AF842763

# Diversity and Cultural Competence in the Health Sector

# Anthropology of Well-Being: *Individual, Community, Society*

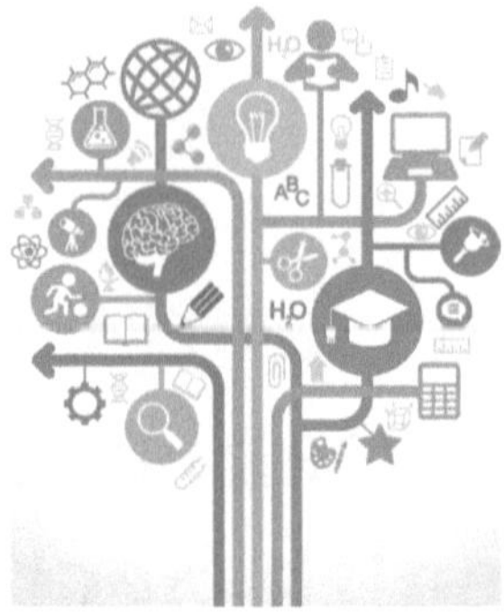

**Series Editor: Ben G. Blount, PhD (SocioEcological Informatics)**

**Mission Statement**

Well-being is central and important in people's daily lives and life history. This book series brings about understanding of what the complex concepts of well-being include. The concepts of quality of life, life satisfaction, and happiness will be explored and viewed at the individual level, the community level, and the level of society. The series encourages and promotes research into the concept of well-being, how it appears to be defined culturally, and how it is utilized across levels and across different social, economic, and ethnic groups. Understandings of how well-being promotes stability and resilience will also be critical to advances in understanding, as well as how well-being can be implemented as a goal in resisting vulnerabilities and in adaptation. Series books include monographs and edited collections by a range of academics, from rising scholars to experts in relevant fields.

**Advisory Board Members**

***Steven Jacob, Kathleen Galvin, Carlos Garcia-Quijano, Cynthia Isenhour, and Richard Pollnac***

**Recent Titles in the Series**

*Diversity and Cultural Competence in the Health Sector: Ebola-Affected Countries in West Africa*, edited by Mohamed Kanu, Elizabeth A. Williams, and Charles Williams

*Everyday Food Practices: Commercialisation and Consumption in the Periphery of the Global North*, by Tarunna Sebastian

*No Perfect Birth: Trauma and Obstetric Care in the Rural United States*, by Kristin Haltinner

*Love and its Entanglements among the Enxet of Paraguay: Social and Kinship Relations within a Market Economy*, by Stephen Kidd

*Care Work and Medical Travel: Exploring the Emotional Dimensions of Caring on the Move*, by Cecilia Vindrola-Padros

# Diversity and Cultural Competence in the Health Sector

## Ebola-Affected Countries in West Africa

Mohamed Kanu, Elizabeth A. Williams,
and Charles Williams

LEXINGTON BOOKS
*Lanham • Boulder • New York • London*

Published by Lexington Books
An imprint of The Rowman & Littlefield Publishing Group, Inc.
4501 Forbes Boulevard, Suite 200, Lanham, Maryland 20706
www.rowman.com

6 Tinworth Street, London SE11 5AL, United Kingdom

Copyright © 2021 by The Rowman & Littlefield Publishing Group, Inc.

*All rights reserved.* No part of this book may be reproduced in any form or by any electronic or mechanical means, including information storage and retrieval systems, without written permission from the publisher, except by a reviewer who may quote passages in a review.

British Library Cataloguing in Publication Information Available

**Library of Congress Cataloging-in-Publication Data**

Names: Kanu, Mohamed, author. | Williams, Elizabeth A., 1972- author. | Williams, Charles, 1946- author.
Title: Diversity and cultural competence in the health sector : Ebola-affected countries in West Africa / Mohamed Kanu, Elizabeth Williams, and Charles Williams.
Description: Lanham : Lexington Books, 2021. | Series: Anthropology of well-being: individual, community, society | Includes bibliographical references and index.
Identifiers: LCCN 2021025177 (print) | LCCN 2021025178 (ebook) | ISBN 9781793645760 (cloth) | ISBN 9781793645777 (ebook)
Subjects: LCSH: Public health—Africa, West. | Public health personnel—Professional ethics—Africa, West. | Cultural competence—Africa, West.
Classification: LCC RA552.W5 K36 2021 (print) | LCC RA552.W5 (ebook) | DDC 362.10966—dc23
LC record available at https://lccn.loc.gov/2021025177
LC ebook record available at https://lccn.loc.gov/2021025178

*This book is dedicated to all those who lost their lives to the Ebola virus, their families, and all the commendable healthcare providers and volunteers for the giving of their sacrificial time and efforts to save lives and eradicate this deadly disease.*

# Contents

# List of Figures and Tables

## FIGURES



## TABLE

# Preface

For ages, infectious or communicable diseases have been part of human existence, and humans and animals (domesticated and wild) have managed to endure the causative agents (viruses, bacteria, etc.) of these diseases. As scientific discovery has evolved and continued to improve, humans have become better adept at managing these sometimes life-threatening organisms whether they are viruses, bacteria or something else.

Global cooperation among nations has become a "forced necessity" because fighting against infectious diseases can be likened to efforts against other threats like terrorism and global warming, in that countries where these problems originate are not the only ones to experience the negative consequences of these diseases. Because of globalization and international travel, which connect the world as a global village, the impact of a deadly infectious disease outbreak in one location reverberates in other faraway countries unless quick and concerted action is taken.

Within the last 25 years, many major infectious disease outbreaks have attracted global attention. A few notable examples include the 1997 H5N1 virus (avian influenza), the 2002 SARS outbreak in China, the Zika virus of 2015 in Brazil, frequent episodes of Ebola in the Democratic Republic of Congo, and the current 2020 COVID-19 pandemic. Although these outbreaks killed many people, the Ebola outbreak of 2014–2016 in West Africa is remembered as the biggest Ebola epidemic to date, claiming over 11,000 lives according to some estimates.

During the 2014 Ebola outbreak, many lessons were learned and have been used to improve health emergency preparedness by strengthening health care delivery and public health systems within the affected countries. By most accounts, the poorly resourced public health systems of the three most affected countries of Sierra Leone, Liberia, and Guinea are better equipped today than they were at the time of the outbreak. Health surveillance systems within these countries have been reinforced, often with the help of development partners and other reputable health organizations and agencies.

At the height of the Ebola outbreak, one of the key lessons learned was understanding cultural practices and their impact on the fight against the highly contagious disease. An expanded notion of that understanding and the need to integrate cultural attributes of a population into infectious disease prevention and treatment strategies are aspects of cultural competency. In this book, we examine the relationship between culture, cultural practices, and their impact on peoples' health behaviors and health system responses during the Ebola outbreak in the three neighboring countries mentioned above, which were the hardest hit in the West African subregion.

The book focuses primarily on Sierra Leone (more than on the other two countries) because Sierra Leone suffered the highest mortality rates among the three countries. The authors used extant literature to develop the chapters, and a survey was conducted among ethnic groups in Sierra Leone to provide primary data about perceptions and use of traditional medical practices before and during the Ebola outbreak.

In the case of the recent COVID-19 pandemic, the fight against this communicable disease has been compounded by an unprecedented level of politicization of the issue (and to some extent fear of vaccines), which has resulted in a high degree of vaccination resistance in some countries. Furthermore, while we applaud the efforts of the World Health Organization and the magnanimity of some developed countries to allocate vaccines to countries with insufficient vaccine supply, the new "vaccine nationalism" where developed countries purchase and/or stock more vaccine supplies than they actually need poses a huge challenge for populations in less developed nations with less access to vaccines.

The fight to prevent the rapid spread of future infectious disease outbreaks and find treatments for emerging and re-emerging diseases will continue to pose challenges across the world. Wealthy and poorer nations will have to collaborate for the world to succeed in addressing infectious diseases. This is because, with infectious diseases, the success of one country is predicated on the success of others. This fight to prevent and control infectious disease outbreaks has to be persistent and sustained. To paraphrase the African novelist Chinua Achebe in his famous book *Things Fall Apart*, he writes that "as long as men have learned to shoot their guns without missing, birds who are targeted will fly without perching." The analogy depicts the relationship between viruses and bacteria on one hand, and scientists, the health industry and national governments, on the other. Each side will adjust to either continue to pose a threat (as the virus does) or work to provide a prevention or treatment response to the threat. The latter is the role of the health industry and its partners (scientists and government, among others).

Infectious or communicable diseases are part of human existence. Communities, governments, scientists, the health industry, and individuals must work together in culturally competent ways to respond to the intermittent threat posed by these ever-present menaces. Behavior, lifestyle, policy, and practice are critical pieces of the disease prevention and control puzzle.

Mohamed Kanu
Professor, Department of Public Health,
Tennessee State University
United States of America.

# Acknowledgments

This book is the product of the hard work and support of many people. First, all the authors thank members of our respective families (wives, children, siblings and grandchildren) for the encouragement they provided to us during the time of writing. Many times, we took away valuable family time from them because we wanted to complete this project on time. In that regard the following people deserve special mention: Mrs. Yeabu Koroma-Kanu, Ms. Anais Bash-Taqi, Dr. Hilda Jane Booker Williams, Rev. Dr. Elizabeth Ann Williams, Charles Christopher Williams, Kylan Isaiah Warren, Brennon Christopher Williams (Mister B), and Arriana Danielle Williams (Ladybug).

Even as co-author of one of the chapters in the book, Ms. Gloria Crawford's contribution to the preparation of supporting documents to the manuscript was phenomenal, and we thank her immensely for that. She also carefully read through the first draft of the manuscript and served as an internal editor.

We acknowledge the patience, encouragement, and timely responses of Kasey Beduhn (acquisitions editor) of Lexington Books, Rowman & Littlefield, during the development of the manuscript. We are very thankful for all of her support and that of other members of her team.

We are also thankful to Professor Mario Azevedo for his scholarship which helped to inspire this publication. His work on the health of Africans since precolonial times to his more recent publications on Ebola and its impact on many parts of Africa served as a source of inspiration for this work.

We owe our colleagues in the Department of Public Health, Health Administration and Health Sciences at Tennessee State University in Nashville, tremendous amounts of appreciation for the various forms of support they provided to some of the authors in the book.

# Introduction

## *The Nexus between Cultural Sensitivity and Health Services*

Mohamed Kanu

For many years, health professionals have crisscrossed the world in service to mankind. In the colonial period, missionary teams were known to make these trips to many parts of Africa to deliver much-needed health services to vulnerable populations in less-resourced communities. Today, health professionals and other technical staff members working for reputable institutions such as the World Health Organization, Centers for Disease Control and Prevention (USA), Médecins Sans Frontières (MSF), or Doctors Without Borders, and many others live and work in countries outside their places of birth. In these foreign job stations, foreign workers deal with local cultural diversity issues, some of which have implications for health. Often, these professionals are at the epicenter of health programs development and implementation. In order to be successful, health programs within and outside Ministries of Health must be designed and delivered in a culturally sensitive manner, if locals will use and adapt them. In an increasingly diverse global community, foreign health experts on whom developing countries heavily depend for technical advice will be hard-pressed to understand some cultural nuances, especially those related to health-seeking behaviors in local communities.

Health programs that are not culturally sensitive risk being shunned by beneficiaries for which they are intended. As a result, it is critical that both local and foreign health professionals understand some basic characteristics of culturally sensitive programming in the health sector. During the 2014–2016 Ebola Outbreak in West Africa, some local cultural practices were found to be inimical to the health of people in many communities. For instance, burial practices constituted a high risk of Ebola virus transmission when relatives of deceased Ebola victims insisted on washing the bodies of dead victims, as a last act of respect and show of affection for departed relatives. Because of this cultural practice, infection spread, and many lives were lost. According to the World Health Organization, nearly 60 percent of all Ebola cases in Guinea were associated with traditional burial practices (Alexander et al. 2014). With such colossal figures, emphasis on and understanding health-related cultural practices that could enhance culturally sensitive health interventions must be prioritized.

The purpose of this book is to use the Ebola outbreak in West Africa as the basis to address the subject of cultural sensitivity in health services provision in Ebola-affected countries in West Africa. The three most affected countries in the Mano River Basin, which include Guinea, Liberia, and Sierra Leone, are the main focus of this book. But even among the three nations, Sierra Leone, which suffered the most fatalities, has received the most emphasis.

Many Ebola outbreaks had occurred in Sub-Saharan Africa prior to the one in West Africa in 2014. As early as 1976, the infamous Ebola outbreak in Zaire (present-day Democratic Republic of the Congo), which is named after a river in that country was the deadliest (Walsh and Johnson 2018), until the 2014 outbreak in West Africa which is now unprecedented in scope and casualty rates. Records show that previous outbreaks were largely confined in rural areas within the countries where they occurred (Walsh and Johnson 2018); however, the West African epidemic affected residents in metropolitan cities and resulted in more than 11,000 deaths within the subregion.

West Africa comprises 17 countries which include Benin, Burkina Faso, Cape Verde, Côte D'Ivoire, Gambia, Ghana, Guinea, Guinea-Bissau, Liberia, Mali, Mauritania, Niger, Nigeria, Saint Helena, Senegal, Sierra Leone, and Togo (see figure I.1). Among these 17 countries, six of them were affected by the March 2014 Ebola outbreak. These countries include Sierra Leone, Liberia, Guinea, Mali, Senegal, and Nigeria. Of the six affected countries, Sierra Leone and its two immediate neighbors of Guinea and Liberia were the most impacted by the Ebola epidemic. Because of that, most of the discussion about the impact of cultural practices on health outcomes is largely limited to those three countries. The book also discusses the broader importance of cultural sensitivity that is necessary in health services provision beyond the scope of the most affected countries by the epidemic.

It is important to mention early that many ethnic groups in West Africa are found in more than one country due to commercial activities, ethnic affinities, and other factors. This is critically important in this discussion because cultural practices among some ethnic groups are essentially

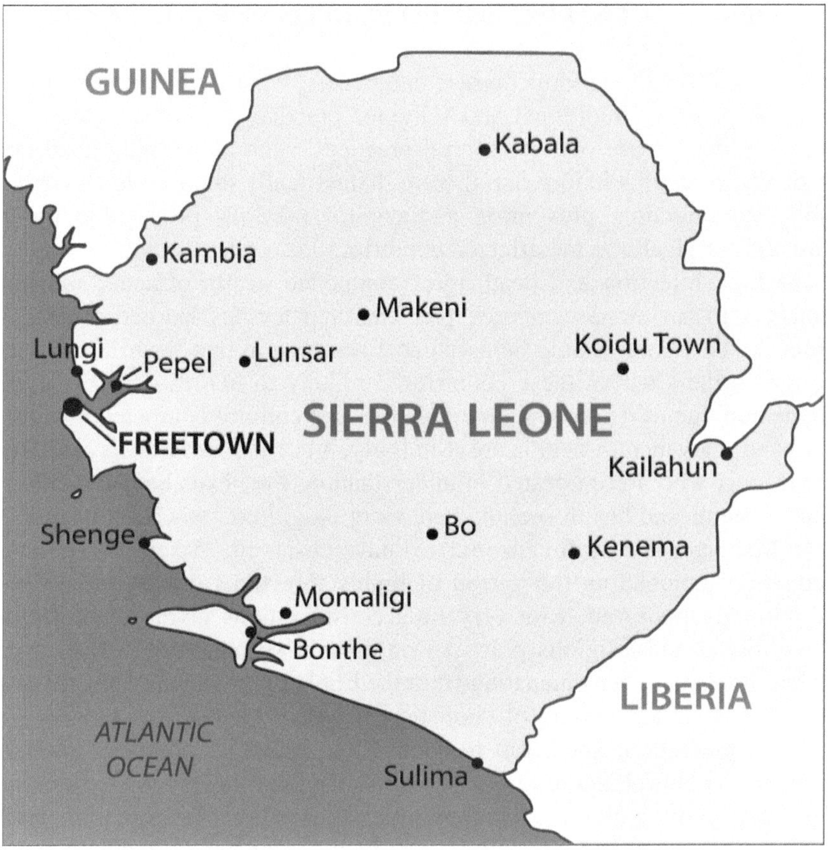


**Figure I.1 Sierra Leone Political Map.** Adobe Stock. *Source:* Adobe Stock, Extended License, Adobe.com, purchased 2021.

the same, regardless of their current country of residence. For example, members of the Fula, Mandingo, and Susu ethnic groups are also found in Guinea, Liberia, Sierra Leone, Mali, Senegal, and other countries within the subregion. The authors of this book surveyed ethnic groups in Sierra Leone regarding health-related cultural beliefs and practices. Because members of some ethnic groups live in more than one country, the authors believe that individuals belonging to the same ethnic group will have identical beliefs and practices even if they live in two different countries within the subregion. To be clear, this is not suggesting that all ethnic groups are essentially the same. Some survey findings are discussed in relevant sections throughout the book.

## DEMAND AND INTENDED PURPOSE OF THE BOOK

During the 2014 Ebola virus disease outbreak in West Africa, it was discovered that peoples' traditional and religious practices exacerbated the rapid spread of the disease, where cultural practices, such as washing dead bodies of Ebola victims before burial were diametrically opposed to the widely publicized infection, prevention and control methods propagated by the Ministries of Health in the affected countries.

The high infection and death rates compelled health officials and policymakers to review documented practices and lessons learned during the outbreak. This book should be a valuable resource in that regard. Local and foreign workers within these countries are likely to find this book a useful companion due to its content on ethnicities and cultural competency models that have relevance in healthcare. Similarly, students, researchers, and general readers who are interested in understanding the nexus between cultural belief systems and health-seeking behaviors should find this book useful.

As Manguvo and Mafuvadze (2015) have observed, "Scientifically-based methods of combatting the spread of highly infectious diseases like Ebola are normally preferred, with very little considerations given to the impact of traditional and religious practices on preventive measures." They argue further that experience emanating from the Ebola outbreak validates the need for a deeper understanding of "holistic contextual factors" (p. 1) alongside scientific methods in the effort to control the spread of infectious diseases. Along with cultural and religious practices, the preponderance of ethnic and cultural diversity within local communities adds another layer of complexity in the social milieu. In Liberia and Sierra Leone, as many as 16 ethnic groups are known to co-exist in each country but each with its different language and cultural practices (Alexander et al. 2014).

From the foregoing paragraphs, it cannot be denied that the 2014 Ebola outbreak exposed the need for a more serious conversation about the impact of cultural and religious practices, and their impact on health promotion and disease prevention. Incidentally, many of the publications focusing on this important subject exist in the form of peer-review journal articles that are largely available to an academically based readership at the expense of the general public. The authors hope this book will be suitable to academics (including students) conducting research, as well as public health practitioners and members of the general public.

The authors of this publication also believe that this book will be a worthy undertaking if reading it either by government officials or policy makers results in developing new policies relating to cultural sensitivity in healthcare; researchers in the assembly of knowledge; civil society activists who advocate for social justice in achieving good health outcomes for citizens;

students who might broaden their knowledge as a result of reading the book; or public health practitioners who might find this book as a useful resource in the practice of public health. To provide the reader some forecast of what to expect, the book is divided into six chapters with an introduction that are described in the following paragraphs.

Introduction: This brief introductory chapter makes the case about why this book is necessary at this time. Basically, this chapter sets the stage with mention of the countries within the West African sub-region that constitutes the setting for the book, and introduces the reader to some basic assumptions on health sector challenges for the region.

Chapter 1 discusses the connection between cultural beliefs, values, practices, and their relationship to health-seeking behaviors and practices. This chapter takes a broad anthropological approach to this subject and draws examples from societies around the world, while focusing mainly on contemporary practices. Specifically, the discussion focuses on critical definitions of culture, ethnomedicine, variation of cultural practices relating to health, and effects of cultural practices on health, with relevance to Sierra Leone. Some survey data of a study introduced in chapter one, are presented in this chapter.

Chapter 2 provides a social context for understanding the concept of multiple ethnicities in West Africa. Using Sierra Leone as a case study, the chapter briefly traces the origins of specific ethnic groups and explores some of their cultural practices and belief systems. Although some of these ethnic groups are also found in other countries within West Africa, this chapter is particularly relevant to readers who are non-natives to the three most Ebola-affected countries of Guinea, Liberia, and Sierra Leone. Furthermore, the chapter sets the stage for a heightened discussion of the social context for a better discussion, and demonstration, of many of the health-related cultural beliefs and practices found among different ethnic groups.

Chapter 3 briefly describes the early presence of Ebola in other parts of Sub-Saharan Africa, outside the West Africa subregion. It then presents the 2014–2016 West African outbreak as a case study to demonstrate the extent to which cultural and religious practices affected the containment of the epidemic. Empirical data are used to demonstrate how cultural practices among some of the ethnic groups presented in the previous chapter aided the spread of the Ebola epidemic. The chapter closes with an exploration of non-cultural-related factors that also facilitated the spread of the epidemic across communities.

Chapter 4 discusses the important concepts of traditional medicine and alternative or complementary medicine with reference to regions of the world where they are prevalent. Based on some of the cultural factors aiding the spread of Ebola in chapter 3, this chapter focuses on necessary steps at standardizing the modus operandi of non-Western traditional healers. Because of the importance of behavioral lifestyles in health promotion and disease prevention, the chapter also discusses behavioral science theories and practice models developed by members of the research community and used in the public health domain.

Chapter 5 focuses on the twin concepts of health disparities and cultural competency among health professionals. The problems of unacknowledged bias based on ethnocentrism and/or other factors could lead to poor quality of healthcare. This chapter discusses different cultural competency models that will help professionals to assess their ability to provide culturally competent health services to their clients. Essentially, the chapter seeks to answer the question, "How can public health and other allied health practitioners use cultural competency skills to provide culturally sensitive services to patients and communities with strong cultural values/ties?"

Chapter 6 offers recommendations based on traditional, religious, and cultural sensitivity practices to improve public health practice. Recommendations are focused on relevant public policy development and public health practitioner guidelines, including the increased role of the Ministry of Health officials, and other stakeholder groupings within the health sector. Consistent with the focus of this book, strong emphasis is placed on the promotion of cultural sensitivity among health professionals to enhance health promotion and disease prevention within the public and private health sectors.

## SOME BASIC ASSUMPTIONS UNDERLYING THE DEVELOPMENT OF THIS BOOK

Sierra Leone and many countries in West Africa are donor-driven and by extension, many health programs receive financial and technical support from international non-governmental organizations, such as the United Nations and its agencies, the World Bank and others such as Doctors Without Borders. Similarly, diplomatic missions and their staff members have provided both financial, as well as technical support to Ministries of Health in Africa at large. For the three countries most affected by the Ebola outbreak, it is undeniable that the epidemic would have lasted much longer were it not for the support of philanthropist individuals, local and international organizations, humanitarian agencies, and foreign governments-led initiatives frequently known as the International Community.

Thanks to help from the aforementioned sources that came to the rescue of the West African countries which were attacked by a deadly virus at a time when they were ill-prepared to launch a strong defense of their people. It has been approximately four years since the Ebola epidemic ended. Before the beginning of the fourth year (2020), after Ebola ended in 2016, the world is again, contending with another pandemic (COVID-19) of unimaginable proportions, claiming hundreds of thousands of lives and devastating global economies.

In West Africa, which was the epicenter of the Ebola epidemic, some of the challenges that existed prior to the outbreak are still present in varying degrees across different countries. One only needs to examine the level of reliance of these countries on developed nations, and its institutions such as the World Bank. Undeniably, some progress has been made through the technical and financial support of donor and local governments in establishing surveillance and other systems to manage health emergencies. In spite of this fact, the authors feel comfortable in making the following assumptions about many of the affected countries by the Ebola epidemic.

## Some Assumptions Applicable to Health Systems in Sub-Saharan Africa

- Even within the relatively small countries across West Africa, variations relating to cultural differences and health-seeking behaviors abound among ethnic groups.
- Closely related to the above, local health practitioners, as well as foreign technical experts in health services delivery, could benefit from cultural sensitivity dialogue and/or training.
- In spite of well-meaning regional proclamations such as the Ouagadougou (Burkina Faso 2008) Declaration calling for African governments to allocate 15 percent of GDP to fund health sectors, many will remain underfunded.
- Corruption will continue to plague the functioning of health systems in many countries in Africa.
- In addition to being underfunded, many health systems will operate at below capacity in terms of human resource capacity.
- The One Health approach which calls for related polices among health ministries is laudable and a step in the right direction; however, the process may be lengthy in developing because many other line ministries are under resourced.
- Health emergencies, both natural and man-made, will occur intermittently and these resource-strapped nations must develop their own local capacity to respond adequately, and cease to heavily rely on developed nations for their rescue.
- To compound the problem of human resource capacity, brain-drain will continue to decimate Africa's human resource pool until significant improvements in service conditions are achieved to slow the pace.

As long as pandemics and epidemics continue to emerge, and the tenets of globalization remain at play (rapid travel, global trade, etc.), the health of the world will be better only when individuals and communities recognize the truth imbedded in the definition of public health by the Institute of Medicine in the United States of America, that "public health is what we, as a society, do collectively to assure the conditions in which people can be healthy" (Institute of Medicine 1998, p. 1).

*Chapter 1*

# The Interface between Cultural Beliefs, Practices, and Health

Charles Williams

## INTRODUCTION: CULTURE ENABLES HUMANS TO ADAPT AND SURVIVE

Most of us are aware that beliefs lead to behaviors, and behaviors lead to consequences, whether positive or negative; however, most of us do not know that it is because of the powerful influence of culture in human life. Therefore, how we view consequences in everyday life shapes both individual and group behaviors and beliefs. Unfortunately, depending solely on consequences to change behaviors, for example, in a health crisis, does not enable the sort of real change that most health professionals imagine when they set out to transform the health of a community. This is because values held by individuals also play a vital role in how people behave. This chapter is intended to provide awareness as well as understanding of the universal relationship between beliefs, values, behavior, and health in the country of Sierra Leone, West Africa. Moreover, it will provide insights into why significant culture transformations in health care and other biomedical efforts appear to progress very slowly.

## HOW CULTURE INFLUENCES HEALTH BELIEFS

Predominantly because of culture and traditions passed from one generation to the next, all human societies—large and small, industrialized and non-industrialized, and developed and undeveloped—have systems of health beliefs and practices to explain what causes illness, how it can be cured or treated, and who should be involved in the process. Therefore, without a doubt, all human societies and cultures have been inquisitive about a particular custom or practice for treating an illness. Such inquisitions include, what was the origin of the illness, or is the illness unique to one's own group? Or, do neighboring groups have the same custom or practice for remedying the illness? Thus, in reality, all human societies have constructed their own unique inquiry based on beliefs and practices, both steeped in culture.

Anthropology, the social and behavioral science discipline, coined the term "culture," and have long debated an appropriate definition for the concept. However, anthropologists generally view culture as one of the unique features that separate man from other forms of life on earth. Only man, or more appropriately, humans, are culture bearing. Defined as learned and shared attitudes, thoughts, values, and behaviors, culture is also inclusive of all man-made material artifacts. Therefore, the 19th-century British anthropologist Edward B. Tylor (1871) combined the aforementioned elements into the first anthropological definition of culture. Tylor's descriptive definition contends that "Culture . . . is that complex whole which includes knowledge, belief, art, law, morals, custom, and any other capabilities and habits acquired by man as a member of society" (Tylor 1920 [1871], p. 1).

For Tylor, anthropology was a "science of culture," a system for analyzing existing elements of human civilization that are socially created rather than biologically inherited. Since Tylor coined the concept of culture, it has become one of the most valuable tools in the toolbox of today's anthropologists, but not before being thoroughly critiqued and scrutinized in the academy of science.

Yet, today some anthropologists criticize the concept of "culture" as an oversimplification, or generalization of being "too inclusive" to adequately capture the way human groups live through time. Since the turn of the century, anthropologists have come to realize that Tylor's descriptive definition of culture has its limitations, and would not apply to all cultures. Anthropologists such as Alfred Kroeber and Clyde Kluckhohn (1952) began to develop a definition of culture that could be applied broadly. They proposed that culture was not simply behaviors that could be described, but that it also included the psychological, social, biological, and material factors. Thus began a focus on the meaning of behavior, not just a description of the behavior itself. Therefore, an integration of Tylor, Kroeber, and Kluckhohn leads to a broader and general definition of culture that can be applied to all groups in society.

Culture has been defined as an umbrella term which encompasses the social behavior and norms found in all human societies, as well as the knowledge, beliefs, arts, laws, customs, capabilities, and habits of the individuals in these groups. However, many anthropologists today would define culture as the shared set of (implicit and explicit) values, ideas, concepts, and rules of behavior that allow a social group to function and perpetuate itself. Another way to understand culture is to view it as the defined patterns of behavior that are common within a particular population of people such as an ethnic group. In essence, the concept of culture is applicable to both human societies at the macro-level and localized ethnic groups at the micro-level.

While the concept of culture sometimes invokes both feelings and thoughts of a higher level of learning, such as being a scholar or intellectual, or being a connoisseur of the fine arts such as Mozart symphony, or admiration for a fine Monet or Picasso, yet, in the popular vernacular of culture, it does often refer to the arts. A person that is cultured has knowledge of and is a patron of the arts; however, a person who observes and is a patron of folk art is equally just as cultured in the eyes of anthropologists. What about Hip Hop culture? It, too, is culture and greatly valued and appreciated by those who participate and enjoy this form of culture. Within anthropology, higher education, the arts (fine and folk), and Hip Hop are all aspects of culture in Western societies. To understand the concept of culture from the perspective of anthropology, one needs to think broader and holistically.

For many years of ethnographic inquiry and comparative studies of many human societies around the world, past and present, practitioners of anthropology have learned that what is common in all of them are its "basic characteristics," or human universals namely, language, social, economic, and political organization, religion, courtship, marriage, childrearing, funerals and games, to name a few.

Culture is the lens through which we see ourselves, others, and the world around us; it is a continuous, human process of learned behavior that is not genetically or biologically transmitted from one member of the group to the next. It is learned over a lifetime through a process known as enculturation. Enculturation is the process by which people learn values and behaviors that are appropriate or necessary in their surrounding culture. Thus, in all human societies, adults teach their youth social roles that must be adhered to for the benefit of the group. Also, as children have learned from their parents and other groups when they become adults, they pass on cultural skills and vital information to the next generation. For example, as stated by Alhaji BMS Turay, a medical herbalist at Connaught hospital in Freetown, Sierra Leone, "I combined my knowledge of plants with traditional healing, which I learned from my mother, who was a healer." Turay, as with most children, learned early in life to imitate and follow the roles played by their parents who serve important roles as educators, ministers, lawyers, and doctors.

Culture is continuously shared among group members at both the macro- and micro-levels of human societies. We may have our own cultural peculiarities within our local or community ethnic group; however, we also share a large part of our culture with others at the societal level. According to the pattern of health care utilization and traditional and complementary medicine use among Ebola survivors in Sierra Leone (2019), the practitioners of traditional and indigenous medicine rely mainly upon medicinal plants and herbs for the preparation of therapeutic substances that are very popular among the people of Sierra Leone. Four years after the Ebola scourge in late March 2014 came to an end, one of the authors, an anthropologist and public health researcher at Tennessee State University, and others conducted a study, entitled "Survey about Traditional Health Beliefs and Practices in Sierra Leone," which also supports the widespread use of traditional and complementary medicine. The study consisted of 500 respondents drawn from mostly urban and peri-urban settlements throughout Sierra Leone. Survey questions ranged from cultural beliefs and practices that potentially exposed people to Ebola infection, causes of Ebola, loss of close and distant relatives, as well as views about post-Ebola survivor community relationships. Therefore, key sources of information about traditional and complementary medicine (T&CM) are family, friends, and local health providers. The correlation between culture and health-seeking behavior is apparent and quite evident among ethnic groups of Sierra Leone.

Culture is looked at as a whole or the group level rather than at personal or individual level. In large complex societies, different ethnic, racial, and class formations are "partial versions of their representative culture." For example, men experience or see issues or problems different from women, such as sports and military activities. Therefore, culture is a complex pool of behavior and knowledge to which various types of people contribute.

Culture is symbolically transmitted from one member of the group to the next through a continuous process of sharing. It assigns meaning and constructs a nomenclature of things in one's daily life. Therefore, the language of any group of people may be the most important representation of the symbolic nature of culture. Language, which can be both verbal and non-verbal, is one of the primary ways that humans communicate with one another.

Lastly, culture is integrated and all-encompassing. It is a roadmap or blueprint for living, informing ourselves and showing others how to respond in any given situation. Think of it as the functioning of the human body. The human body is composed of 11 mechanistic systems, including the circulatory, respiratory, digestive, excretory, nervous, and endocrine systems. It also includes the immune, integumentary, skeletal, muscle, and reproductive systems. These systems work together to maintain a functioning human body. Culture is also a system, a system of institutions that work together to meet the needs of the group.

Culture is also defined by the extent to which a people perceive information and knowledge about a particular illness and behave based on that information. In this instance, information and knowledge have cultural relevance not only for individuals but also for each member of their group, which can have a profound effect on the group's receptivity to information provided and their willingness to use it. For example, and as previously stated by Alhaji BMS Turay, in reference to his mother, "I combined my knowledge of plants with traditional healing, which I learned from my mother, who was a healer."

Complex industrialized societies, such as the United States, which see disease as a result of natural scientific phenomena, rely almost totally on trained physicians and medical science for treatments to combat microorganisms or use sophisticated technology to diagnose and treat disease. Other societies, such as Sierra Leone, believe illness is the result of supernatural phenomena and promote prayer or other spiritual interventions that counter the presumed disfavor of powerful forces. Therefore, culture plays a major role in a sick person's view of an illness and, of course, their compliance. As Alhaji BMS Turay further contends, "the majority of people [in Sierra Leone] still go to traditional healers, because this was all we initially had" (Obermueller 2012). However, as indicated by the 2020 study mentioned earlier, there is a strong correlation between tradition and complementary medicine across each indicator of age, gender, and education; over 83 percent of respondents in the study with minimal to formal education believe in the efficacy of traditional healers.

The universality of culture, which permeates every cognitive fiber of our being as humans, is not a word or a thing that can easily be defined in any of the world's parlance languages. It is an abstraction or cognitive construct that is worthy of discussion in a broader sense to truly understand the interface between cultural beliefs, practices, and health as defined by the Swiss psychologist Jean Piaget. Cognitive-construction purports that people construct their own understanding and knowledge of the world through their experiences and their reflections upon these experiences (see figure 1.1). In a "What Is Culture?" interview with Kim Ann Zimmermann, Live Science Contributor, July 13, 2017, Cristina De Rossi, anthropologist at Barnet and Southgate College, London, succinctly described culture as encompassing "religion, food, what we wear, how we wear it, our language, marriage, music, what we believe is right or wrong, how we sit at the table, how we greet visitors, how we behave with loved ones, and a million other things." When teaching anthropology at the University of Memphis in Memphis, Tennessee, for 36 plus years, I would constantly tell my students, both graduates and undergraduates, that culture was in their brains as displayed by The Wheel of Culture.

We live, work, play, sleep, and eat our culture on a daily basis, every minute and hour of the day, and every month of the year. We are a walking

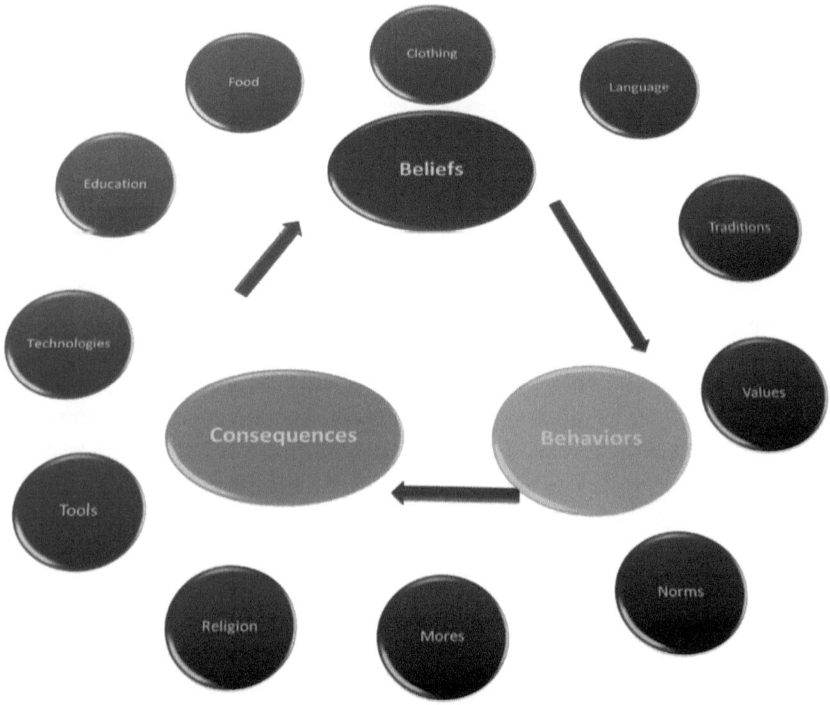


**Figure 1.1 The Wheel of Culture.** Designed by Charles Williams and Gloria Crawford. *Source:* The Wheel of Culture. Designed by Charles Williams and Gloria Crawford.

and talking exhibit of our culture, and there is not much we or anyone else can do about it. Therefore, all living human beings regardless of their ethnicity, humanity, station in life, or their intersectionality are perfect individual culture machines.

In practically all human groups, large and small, complex and noncomplex, there is a belief that has been passed down from generation to generation that a "Creator God" or supernatural intercedes directly or indirectly in our daily lives. According to the Judeo-Christian belief, in the beginning, God created the heaven and the earth, and it was God who created man to have dominion over the fish of the sea, over the fowl of the air, over the cattle, over all the earth, and over every creeping thing that creepeth upon the earth (Genesis 1: 1-26). However, for the multiple ethnic groups that make up the West African country of Sierra Leone—Mende, Temne, Limba, Krio, Fula, Mandingo, Kissi, Kono, Susu, Kru, Kuranko Sherbro, Loko, Yalunka, and others—there is no clear division of people and cultures (Middleton 1997, p. 85). Though details may vary from one ethnic group to another, the general characteristics of traditional beliefs and practices are similar. They all share the concept of "a Creator God who is omnipotent and timeless," but may believe in other deities (multiple supernatural beings). He is also remote from men and does not judge them; nevertheless, it is on this concept that Christian and Muslim missionaries transplant their ideas of God.

All ethnic and cultural groups of Sierra Leone believe that God is the ultimate creator of the material and nonmaterial world. They seldom, however, address him directly in prayer. More genuinely involved in the affairs of the living are thought to be a variety of spirits. Communication between their world and the visible world is provided by dreams, divination, and omens. Closest and most intimate are the spirits of dead ancestors who are believed to participate in the affairs of the living and to be able to help by direct action or by carrying prayers to God. They are greatly respected as the source and guardians of all knowledge. They are approached through sacrifice and invocation by the head of the family.

As stated by Olukoju (2006), "Beliefs include the conviction that there are deep and hidden things about an individual that only diviners, priests, [traditional healers] and other qualified persons can unravel, and presupposes that whatever exists or happens in the physical realm has foundations in the spirit world." However, with over several centuries of being exposed to Europeans and Western education, many people of Sierra Leone, especially the young, mobile, and educated, are becoming more open to contemporary and modern medical treatment. In the 2020 study, when respondents were asked, "Do you believe in the healing power of either: a) Clinical medicine only (pills, injections, etc.), b) Traditional healers/medicine only, c) Fortune tellers/sorcerer, d) Moray-man (use of charms, etc.), and e) Prayers," overwhelmingly, 98.8%, 586 of 593 respondents answered this question. On a related survey, respondents were asked: "When you feel sick, which of the following do you use to treat your illness? Please circle all that applies: a) Clinical or prescription medicine only (pills, injections etc.), b) Traditional practitioner/medicine (herbalist, traditional healers etc.), c) Both clinical and traditional, d) None of the above (please specify)," their responses were as follows: a) Clinical or prescription medicine only (pills, injections etc.), 77.74%; b) Traditional practitioner/medicine (herbalist, traditional healers, etc.), 24.62%; c) Both clinical and traditional, 24.96%; and d) None of the above (please specify), 1.01%. These data clearly support two very important assumptions: 1) Sierra Leoneans, especially the young and better educated, are accepting of modern and clinical medicine and 2) the impact of the Ebola epidemic has shown Sierra Leoneans the efficacy of modern and clinical medicine and the impact of Western healthcare practices.

Middleton (1997) and others further convey that the ethnic groups of Sierra Leone share much more than the cultural notion of a "Creator God"; they also share lineage use rights in land, animal husbandry, and initiations that define role, status, and gender differences, which are informed by belief in an ongoing conflict between benevolent and malevolent forces. Each ethnic group defines itself through situational and contextual articulations of myth, ancestors, and land, a hierarchy of belief, the influence of Islam or Christianity, and access to technology, as well as through Western education and connections to national government (Middleton 1997, p. 86).

Today, and globally, examples abound that illustrate various ways in which human groups believe that "a Creator God, or the Supernatural" has equipped them with the marvelous potential to adapt—within the limits of a created kind—in ways that allow them to pioneer and engage with the dynamics of the earth's constantly changing environments. Each example provides yet another way to understand the creative genius of humans, by way of their culture to successfully survive in almost any environment. For example, in an interview on Weekend Edition Saturday with Shannon Francis, a member of the Hopi Tribe and Navajo Nation, it was revealed that her ancestors' beliefs helped shape her thoughts on the Coronavirus pandemic. According to Francis,

> My grandpa and his grandpa recorded a lot of the genealogy and tracked families through other pandemics such as the flu, influenza, and tuberculosis. That knowledge is always passed down from, you know, mother to daughter, father to son, elder to grandchild. Some of our teachings that I was brought up with is that when in times of other pandemics, everybody would have to kind of go into seclusion, go into their homes, and especially during the winter, it's a time of quiet and reflection and peace. (Shannon Francis, interview by Scott Simon, NPR, Washington, DC, March 28, 2020 7:59 AM ET)

Further, Francis contends that

> My mother said that this is a good thing, because Mother Earth is getting a break from humans—from mining, development, digging her up, you know, her soil, and so this is sort of a break for her. And the natural world is going to restore her, and really, you know, start the healing. (Shannon Francis, interview by Scott Simon, NPR, March 2020)

Yet, as Shannon Francis of the Hopi people, Kadiatu Bangura of Sierra Leone, conveys in another interview with Isabel Coello, a Regional Information Officer for West Africa, ECHO, how she got infected with Ebola, and its impact on her family and community. Before 32-year-old Kadiatu Bangura got infected with Ebola, she was a strong and determined headmaster with six children and a school of 375 students in Kambia, Sierra Leone. When the Ebola epidemic struck her country and schools were closed, she volunteered with other women to inform the communities about how Ebola spreads and what measures are to be taken in order to stop the transmission of the disease (Kadiatu Bangura, interview by Isabel Coello, Regional Information Officer for West Africa, ECHO, 2015).

Unfortunately, Kadiatu contracted the virus from her supervisor who spent the night at her home. The following day, the supervisor left to visit a village nearby, but was sick. The next day, he died and was tested positive for the Ebola virus disease. Almost immediately, Kadiatu was visited by a doctor from the World Health Organization (WHO) and told that she had to be quarantined. She, along with her children, was quarantined, and on the seventh day, Kadiatu began to feel pain in her joints. She called the doctor from WHO, and was immediately carried to an International Medical Corps (IMC) treatment center. As soon as she arrived and received treatment and further testing, the third day, Kadiatu was told that she was tested positive for Ebola.

Treated in a health clinic with biomedicines, operated by IMC, and funded by the European Commission to help fight the outbreak in West Africa, Kadiatu survived Ebola. With recovered strength and passion, Kadiatu now believes that survivors have a role to play in the eradication of Ebola. She wants to share her experience of how she was taken to the clinic and how she was healed. Now Kadiatu states emphatically,

> We [survivors] are examples for other people, and we should pass on our stories because some still do not believe the Ebola exists. That is why they still practice family burial rituals that involve washing the bodies of the dead, a practice that carries a high risk of transmission of the deadly virus. (Kadiatu Bangura, interview by Isabel Coello, Regional Information Officer for West Africa, ECHO, 2015)

Other insights garnered from Kadiatu's interview are as follows: 1) The majority of Sierra Leoneans are afraid of Western medical practices offered in local health clinics, because they think they are killing centers, and 2) Out of fear and ignorance, people are passing wrong information to their relatives concerning the medicines prescribed, the food and drink served to patients, and the overall care of doctors and nurses.

In a 2015 Valley News article by Hongoltz-Hetling entitled "When Science, Faith Clash: In Sierra Leone, a Deadly Gap Between Ritual and Medical Practices," it is reported that

> When the Ebola epidemic swept through the region, killing about 3,900 Sierra Leoneans, one of the dominant storylines that emerged in international coverage spotlighted people who resisted treatment. Many Americans shook their head

> disapprovingly at media reports of patients fleeing hospitals, villagers stoning ambulances, and families persisting in burial rituals that involved washing the bodies of the dead, a practice that carries with it a high risk of transmission of the deadly virus.

This article further conveys that

> few outsiders understood that the underlying cause of those events was not ignorance. Instead, experts say, people fled treatment because of a wide culture gap. The wider cultural gap was throughout Sierra Leone and much of West Africa and evident in the remote Dorma Village of Sierra Leone, where some of the poorest people in the world spend most of their day struggling to feed their families, [and confront the deadly Ebola virus], the witch doctor's power over life and death was well known.

Whether Christian or Muslim "More than 90 percent of Sierra Leoneans believe that traditional demons and spirits are often responsible for everyday events, whether it's a lucky find by a diamond miner, a chronic pain in the back, or a miscarriage" (Hongoltz-Hetling 2015).

As the Navoho Nation, Sierra Leone too is culturally unique and, at the same time, one of Africa's poorest and least healthy countries. In terms of available healthcare and health status, Sierra Leone is very poorly rated. Globally, infant and maternal mortality rates remain among the highest. The major causes of illness within the country are preventable with modern technology and medical advances. Most deaths within the country are attributed to nutritional deficiencies, lack of access to clean water, pneumonia, diarrheal diseases, anemia, malaria, tuberculosis, and HIV/AIDS. Overall health inequalities and recent global infections, such as Ebola, reflect a legacy of poverty and civil wars since gaining independence in 1961 from Great Britain. Applying perspectives from both cultural anthropology and medical anthropology offer a more in-depth understanding of health and illness to intensive praxis to address specific health disparities.

Currently, work in Sierra Leone has adopted a participatory engagement framework with two specific goals: 1) utilizing the disciplines of cultural anthropology, medical anthropology, and public health among a broad coalition of researchers, policymakers, service providers, and grassroots partners to improve health conditions, and 2) engaging community stakeholders' input in, as well as direct governance over, the scope and direction of healthcare system change. Key examples are also presented to illustrate this transformation philosophy and the process of participatory engagement in Sierra Leone.

## THE CATALYTIC CONVERTERS OF CULTURE: BELIEFS AND VALUES

In the context of culture, a belief system is an ideology or set of principles that helps an individual to understand his/her everyday reality. This could be in the form of religion, political affiliation, philosophy, spirituality, or health, as well as many other things. These beliefs are often passed down from generation to generation and are shaped and influenced by various factors such as family, friends, teachers, and environment. Contingent on an individual's circumstances and experiences, beliefs can develop quickly or slowly and play a large role in one's behavior. For example, an individual who has never encountered Western medicine but has utilized traditional healers with effective health care are much more likely to believe in traditional medicine than modern or clinical medicine. Individual beliefs tend to be substantiated first by trust, then by facts, circumstances, and experience. Culture is dynamic and is inevitably subject to some form of change over time; beliefs can be changed by the introduction of new facts, changing circumstances, and evolving experience.

Unlike beliefs, one's values (often referred to as "core values") are deeply rooted in culture and reflect that what one feels is important and essential in their life, or one's principles or standards of behavior. For example, one's values could include concepts such as caring, empathy, or trust, among many others. Individual values are usually reinforced by group or community values such as collectivism and respect for the elderly. For example, a core value of Sierra Leoneans, and conceptualized in an African proverb says: "Those who respect the elderly pave their own road toward success." Children are taught to be respectful to elders and revere them for their experience, their wealth of knowledge, and their role as significant stakeholders in society. They are considered the custodians of the culture. In Sierra Leone, specifically, and Africa generally, the elderly customarily live with their children or relatives where all their financial, medical, and emotional needs are met. Unlike in the West, it is seen as a shameful act for one's aged parents to be taken to a home for the elderly while their children are still alive. However, as a result of the 11-year brutal civil war in Sierra Leone, this cherished family ethos was disrupted and left in its wake a growing neglect of the poor and elderly. Unfortunately, this is another example of a culture changing, but with negative effects.

Also, in cultural groups, there are individual and group values which often overlap or even become indistinguishable. For example, the secret Poro societies of West Africa, introduced by Mande migrants to the region during 1000 AD, are now an integral part of the life and culture of Sierra Leone (Fyfe 1979). The Poro society consists of two affiliated and secret associations—one for men and one for women—that are responsible for organizing the initiations that prepare boys and young men and girls and young women for adult life. Aldridge (1901) contends that Poro represents a type of fraternal society and governs the entire native with its code of laws. However, Olukoju (2006) indicates that Poro society, for both elite and non-elite, is characterized by a predisposition toward secrecy ("do not speak it") and an ingrained belief in the intervention of mysterious forces in human affairs. Germane to cultural and group values toward health held by the people of Sierra Leone, they are intrinsically linked to Poro requirements and dictates as by various studies (Aldridge 1901; Fyfe 1979; Olukoju 2006).

Unfortunately, what should be viewed as a positive, should be the common ground between individual and group values in developing parts of the world is where health crises (epidemics and pandemics) have been devastating. For example, the Ebola epidemic in Sierra Leone and Liberia and the COVID-19 pandemic among the Navaho people in the southwestern United States. Therefore, the opportunity to change a given cultural group depends almost exclusively on understanding individual and group values which ultimately define standards of behavior. Because culture is the collection of expectations and norms that determine how a group behaves; values, behavior, and culture are inseparable.

To learn of the health-related beliefs, knowledge, and practices of a cultural group is known as ethnomedicine and the primary goals of medical anthropology. How do cultures understand the concepts of health and illness? Are there cultural knowledge and beliefs about what causes illness? How does knowledge and beliefs impact the treatment of illness? Is there a therapeutic process for illness? Are there individuals who specialize in the therapeutic process, and what are their practices for remedying illness? Are there special therapies, and how are they administered? These are some questions asked by medical anthropologists in the study of ethnomedicine—the study or comparison of the traditional medicine based on bioactive compounds in plants and animals and practiced by various ethnic groups, especially those with little access to Western medticines, for example, indigenous peoples. Its research is interdisciplinary and synonym for traditional medicine.

## IMPACT OF CULTURE ON HEALTH

Unlike illness, which is associated with psychological, cultural and physical factors and tied to an individual's worldview, disease is a verifiable pathogenic condition, or in some cases, psychological or spiritual factors, and tied to an individual's worldview, "health" is culturally specific, subjective, and with no universal definition. Nevertheless, international organizations such as

WHO in its global reach attempted, in 1946, to construct a definition of health that would be amenable to all its global communities. It defines health as "a state of complete physical, mental and social well-being and not merely the absence of disease or infirmity." Although the definition was welcomed by some as being innovative, it was also criticized as being vague, excessively broad, and not construed as measurable. For a long time, it was set aside as an impractical ideal and most discussions of health returned to the practicality of the biomedical model. Having developed a definition of health, WHO's aim was to apply laudable standards for achieving good health and recognize that cultural factors undergird this concept (Miller 2011).

Health is a cultural concept because it is framed and shaped by culture, our perception of the world (worldview), and our individual personal experiences. In conjunction with other social determinants of health and disease, such as income and social status, culture helps one to understand the following:

- The view of health and illness by patients and health providers.
- The interaction between patient and health care providers. For example, not making direct eye contact is a sign of respect in many cultures, but a care provider may wonder if the same behavior means her patient is depressed.
- The views about disease causation from the perspective of patients and health providers are often quite different. For example, in many cultures, patients are not familiar with the Western germ theory and may instead believe in religious supplication, magic fatalism, or demonic spirits. They may not accept a diagnosis and may even believe in predestination (they cannot change the course of events and instead, they can only accept circumstances as they unfold).

There are several diseases that are stigmatized: mental disorders, AIDS, venereal diseases, leprosy, certain skin diseases, and now, Ebola and COVID-19. People with these diseases, practically the world over, are discriminated in the health care system; they usually receive much less social support than those who have non-stigmatizing illnesses and, what is possibly worst, they have grave difficulties in organizing their lives if their disease has caused an impairment that can lead to disability and handicaps.

- The expressed experience of illness and pain. In Sierra Leone as a result of Ebola, abdominal pain followed by joint pain and back pain were the most cited post-Ebola indications for T&CM use (Wardle et al. 2019).
- The when, where, why, and how patients seek health care (whether from an allied health care provider or a medical doctor) when a problem becomes severe.
- The degree of understanding and compliance with treatment options recommended by health care providers who do not share their cultural beliefs.

Conversely, the influences of culture on health are vast and often unimaginable because it affects perceptions of health, illnesses and death, beliefs about causes of disease, approaches to health promotion, how illness and pain are experienced and expressed, where patients seek help, and the types of treatment patients prefer.

The role that culture plays in health and illness interactions and influences are enormous. How an individual might view an illness or treatment affects how a health practitioner should address their patient; for example, patient as a child vs patient as an elderly person, or as mentioned earlier, people in some cultures, as some Sierra Leoneans, believe illness is the will of a higher power and may be more reluctant to receive health care.

## INTERSECTIONALITY OF HEALTH AND ILLNESS

There is an increasing number of studies which shows the need and capacity of humans throughtout the world that seek to understand the difference between health and illness. This cultural information at both the individual and group levels is essential for survival, and even among school-age children. Several studies (Natapoff 1982; Burbach and Peterson 1986; Rice 1994; Piko and Bak 2006) indicate that school children have considerable knowledge about health, illness, and disease risks. According to WHO, health is a state of complete physical, mental, and social well-being and not the absence of disease. Health awareness, taught to children in a variety of ways, mostly by parents and teachers, account for their high level of health-consciousness and generally held positive attitudes toward health. Many children are knowledgeable of the biomedical approach to health, but at the same time, they are aware of holistic views of health as well. Their experiences (e.g., childhood illness and infections) and their social and cultural environment also play an important role in how children conceptualize the concepts of health and illness.

Health is an ordinary state of being; however, illness is inclusive of the following:

- An impairment of normal physiological functioning affecting part, or all of an organism
- Poor health resulting from disease of body or mind, sickness
- The state of being unwell
- Sickness and synonym with illness
- Evil wickedness
- An abnormal condition of a body part, organ, or system of an organism resulting from various causes such as infection, inflammation, or genetic defects and illness, is negative, whereas health is viewed as positive

Overall health conditions in West Africa, in particular Sierra Leone, have never been equal to health conditions in the Western world for a variety of reasons, and too extensive to discuss in this writing. However, Africa, the birthplace of humankind, and its health conditions are equally as important, and deserving of equal attention and respect from the global community of scientists and health professionals. Therefore, two immediate questions are, what accounts for Africa's health disparities, and what is the most credible answer? Today's viral diseases such as Ebola, Influenza A (H1N1), SARS, MERS, Zika virus, and most recently COVID-19 are not respectful of national and international borders and boundaries, or the intersectionality of race, class, age, and gender. History tells us that many of the aforementioned diseases are old world diseases and have overwhelmed Africa for many centuries, for example Influenza A. The Influenza Pandemic killed 1,072 people in Sierra Leone within five weeks beginning in mid-August 1918, when a ship with infected sailors docked in its port before spreading to Gambia, Senegal, and other West African countries (Potter 2001).

Prior to the advent of the Europeans and African colonization, as early as 1830 in North Africa (Mostyn and Hourani 1988), in particular, West Africa in the 1880s (Porter 2015), some of the major presenting illnesses or health problems were maternal healthcare, such as the dangers of childbirth, and infectious diseases like malaria, pneumonia, diarrhea, HIV, and tuberculosis. All were under the control of culture and local religious and herbal practitioners, or traditional medicine (folk medicine, indigenous medicine, healing and shamanism).

Traditional medicine was offered by an array of practitioners known as collective as "traditional healers," including diviners, midwives, and herbalists. These gatekeepers provided the dominant healthcare for millions of people in Africa prior to the arrival of the Europeans and science-based biomedicine (Abdullahi 2011). According to Helwig 2005, traditional healers found medical cures for a variety of illnesses including cancer, psychiatric disorders, high blood pressure, cholera, most venereal diseases, epilepsy, asthma, eczema, fever, anxiety, depression, benign prostatic hyperplasia, urinary tract infections, gout, and healing of wounds and burns and even Ebola (Traditional African medicine, Gale Encyclopedia of Alternative Medicine, Retrieved October12, 2020).

The hand in glove analogy (an agreement or relationship between things otherwise different) is appropriate here to describe the relationship between the all-encompassing concept of culture and one of its essential components, health. By far, health which includes so many key aspects of culture (the physical, social, emotional, spiritual, and perceptional) is one of its key components because of its vital necessity for human survival. For humans to maintain good health and a quality of well-being, they must recognize all aspects of health and keep them in balance so that they work best for the individual and the group. Health is a condition in which all the given aspects work in a holistic way. Body, mind, spirit, family, friends, community, education, job, and beliefs determine the health of a person.

The Wheel of Health (WOH), created by Duke Integrative Medicine in 2010, is a visual reminder of the many different layers of one's whole life and health. All of the areas that are included in the WOH can affect health and have connections to one another.

The objective here is to argue the relationship between culture and health and its appendages. As I would inform students, the glove/health analogy cannot do anything by itself, but with the hand as representative of culture and inside of the glove, it could become functional, move, and provide some kind of valuable utilitarian service.

By way of a brief explanation of WOH and its integral and complex relationship with culture, the three colors of the Wheel (yellow, green and blue) represent the following:

- Yellow: At the center of WOH is the individual whose values, goals, and needs determine the course of their life.
- Green: Surrounding the individual at the center of WOH is self-help and self-care and choices made to improve the state of health acquired mainly through learned cultural knowledge and information (enculturation).
- Blue: Other supports which could include knowledge and practices provided by traditional healers or biomedical practitioners. These are interventions sought by an individual when self-help and self-care therapies are ineffective. The objective here is "staying healthy," whether that includes prevention or treatment.

In order to understand the complexities and nuances of culture and health, Duke Integrative Medicine model of care, which advocates for both conventional and complementary therapies, is ideal. Therapies and services from a Western perspective would include physicians, nurses, nutritionists, and other conventional health care workers, as well as integrative health coaches, acupuncturists, massage therapists, psychologists, mind-body therapists, and a wide range of other complementary health care providers. However, from a traditional perspective, it includes shamans, curandero's, diviners, herbalists, midwives or traditional birth attendants, traditional surgeons, or any type of folk healers.

Given that health is not only the absence of an ailment or disease but also the complete physical, mental, emotional, social, and spiritual well-being of a person, good health and well-being should be the goal of all health practitioners, whether they dispense biomedical therapies or traditional folk-medicines and are appropriate for the cultures they are found. The yardstick of measurement as to their efficacy must involve three key aspects of quality healthcare that is patient-centered, such as:

- Care should be accessible and relied on or trusted, depending on achievement, accuracy, honesty, and so on.
- Provide patients with clear, concise, but culturally relevant and comprehensible information concerning their condition and regiment of care.
- Provide patients with emotional support, respect, and empathy throughout the regiment of care.
- Involve patients in the decision-making process, one of the most important aspects of quality care.
- Encourage and provide support for patients' self-care in conjunction with compliance.
- Effective treatment must be individualized to meet multiple needs of the patient and include their socio-psychological and cultural needs.

## *Chapter 2*

# Ethnic Groups of Sierra Leone

Regina Bash-Taqi and Gloria J. Crawford

This chapter describes the different ethnic groups in Sierra Leone, and some of their health-related cultural beliefs and practices. There are originally 18 ethnic groups in Sierra Leone, but only a few of them have struggled to retain their own identities and have been merged into some of the larger ones (Alie 2016). In spite of this ethnic distinction, many health-related cultural beliefs and practices frequently extend across ethnic lines. To provide a context for understanding these practices, many of the ethnic groups are briefly described, along with some of their basic characteristics and belief systems. To reiterate, ethnic groups from the other West African countries, affected by Ebola, are not included; however, some of the ethnic groups discussed in this chapter (e.g., the Fula, the Mandingo, and the Susu) are often resident in more than one country in the subregion. Therefore, characteristics and practices of these groups are similar regardless of the country where they reside.

## FULA

The Fula are the sixth largest ethnic group in Sierra Leone with 266,581 members and account for 3.8 percent of the total population, according to the 2015 national census data in Sierra Leone. In neighboring Guinea, they are the largest. It is critical to mention that this ethnic group is found in almost every country in the West African subregion and beyond, largely due to their involvement in commercial activities. Evidence drawn from the Fulani oral tradition suggests that this group of people may have originated from Jordan or even farther east (Skutsch 2005). There is also evidence that suggests the Fula of Sierra Leone may draw their origins from the meeting of ancient West

African with North African populations, such as the Berbers and Egyptians (Ndukwe 1996).

Most members of this ethnic group are believed to be Muslims. Being Muslim, they annually fast for one month, which is called the month of Ramadan. The Fula pray five times a day, and study their religious book, the Qur'an/Koran. It cannot be denied that a minority of them might belong to other faiths such as Christianity.

Music and Art are a big part of the cultural practices of the Fula, and the musical repertoire includes drums, horns, and flutes. Other common cultural practices include circumcisions at age seven—for the young men, introducing them into the world as herders or farmers, naming ceremonies and even arranged marriages (Countries and Their Cultures, Fulani). Dress codes vary among the Fulani people; however, both men and women who are married dress according to the Islamic tradition, with men wearing large gowns, trousers, and caps; women wear blouses and wraps. Married women wear veils when they go outside of their house. However, nomadic Fulani do not dress as eloquent, and the women do not wear veils (Countries and Their Cultures, Fulani).

Being a nomadic people, there is an added layer of difficulty for the public health system to reach Fulani communities. The Fulani's inclination toward seeking help depends largely on the nature of the disease; for example, if the illness is related to a body part below the waist, many will consider it as a fruit of not following Fulani tradition, making it harder for them to seek help (Gordon 2000). Among the 44 people of the Fula ethnic included in the survey, 20 percent expressed belief in traditional medicine, and 34 percent in prayers as a means of healing. Moreover, 100 percent believe that the practice of washing dead bodies is an important cultural or religious practice that must be followed, emphasizing the highly entrenched cultural and religious beliefs of people in this ethnic group.

## KISSI

The Kissi are believed to have originated from the upper Niger; they were attacked by the Kuranko and pushed further into the interior of the country. They originally settled in Kissy near Freetown in Sierra Leone in 1816 (Gordon 2000) but live in the eastern part of the country close to the border with Guinea. In total, there are well over 890,000 Kissi distributed throughout Western Africa. In Sierra alone, there are 175,000 Kissi people, approximately 2 percent of the country's population (Statistics Sierra Leone 2017).

Although Christianity, as a faith, is steadily growing among the Kissi, most still practice their people's ancestral faith. This belief system entails the role of ancestral spirits as mediators between them and their creator, God. These spirits are often represented as stone statues, to which the village headman prays and offers sacrifice (Joshua Project 2020). Kissi people live in small communities across the forests of Guinea along Sierra Leone and Liberia (Encyclopedia Britannica). The Kissi diet consists of rice, yams, groundnuts, bananas, melons, and taro.

In the current study, many respondents from this ethic group expressed belief in both traditional healers and biomedicine. Seventeen percent also mentioned praying and spiritual healing as ways to deal with health issues. There was also a smaller group of 3 percent (of the 12 respondents) who declared their belief in the services of moray-man and the use of charms to avoid or treat illness.

## KONO

This group today is the fourth largest ethnic group in the country with a little over 361,000 (Statistics Sierra Leone 2017). The Kono people are descendants of the Mali-Guinean people. They settled in the Kono District of Sierra Leone in the 16th century.

The Kono people are mainly farmers, growing rice, cassava, and many other fruits and vegetables. Some Kono people mine diamonds. Much like other ethnic groups of Sierra Leone, Kono men wear full buttoned gowns dyed in lively colors, and often paired with a Kufi hat or fez (Little 1949). The main components of the average Kono diet are rice, cassava, corn, beans, groundnuts, sweet potato, peppers, greens, potato leaf, and cassava leaf. Among the 12 respondents who took part in the survey, 69 percent expressed preference for biomedicine or clinical medicine compared to services of traditional healers; 8 percent mentioned the efficacy of prayer in combating illness.

## KRIO

The Krio people are descendants of former enslaved Africans who fought in the American War of Independence for the British in exchange for the promises of freedom. In 1783, after the war, they were sent to Sierra Leone in Africa (Fyfe 1964). The Krio ethnic group make up approximately 2 percent of Sierra Leone's population. The majority of the Creoles are Christians and a significant number of them are Muslims. Based on their history of early Western exposure and interactions with other local ethnic groups, they developed their native language, which is a mixture of English, indigenous

West African languages, and other European languages. Not surprisingly, all 19 respondents in our survey from this ethnic group expressed belief in, and preference only for biomedicine and no other traditional healing method.

## KRU

There are only 6,000 members of the Kru ethnic group in Sierra Leone (Statistics Sierra Leone 2015). The Kru are predominantly Christian, specifically, Roman Catholic, with a small number of evangelicals (People Groups 2020). Kru is the main language spoken by the Kru people, and they moved to the country from present-day Liberia where many of them still live (Alie 2016). Historically, The Kru are known for their resistance to being taken into slavery. During the Transatlantic Slave Trade, they would resist capture to the extent of taking their own lives to evade surrender. Ceremonies of gift giving maintain a bond among the Kru. There are other rituals performed by their spiritual authorities known as Deya for medical and spiritual healing.

The main staple is rice, which is often flavored with various sauces and spices, and meat or fish as garnishments. On health-seeking behaviors, historically, the Kru have manifested a preference for traditional treatments of illness due to a range of factors, from the belief that certain conditions are spiritual in nature, to the ready availability of a traditional healer in the village (Grepin Mathieu Ashley 2020); however, a lot of this has changed due to exposure to biomedicine.

## KURANKO

As the fifth largest ethnic group with 313,384 members (Statistics Sierra Leone 2017), the Kuranko are a branch of the Malinke tribe that immigrated to Sierra Leone from Guinea. Kuranko people can be found across northeastern Sierra Leone to southern Guinea. The majority of the Kuranko people follow their traditional beliefs; however, some are known to be Muslims. Many live in the Koinadugu district in the north of the country. Literacy and education are helping to change this culture. The Kuranko are reported to be less receptive to seek medical help from outside their own people (Ross 1991).

Constituting the fifth largest ethnic group in Sierra Leone, understanding cultural practices among members of this group is important in improving health care through cultural sensitivity. In a subsample of 25 respondents, 20 percent of them expressed confidence in traditional healing methods.

## LIMBA

The exact origin of the Limba is difficult to trace; however, it is believed they settled in Sierra Leone by the 8th century (Fyle 1982). According to the Sierra Leonean historian Joe A.D. Alie (2016), this group claims no tradition of movement from any other regions of the world into Sierra Leone, and have always been natives of Sierra Leone. They are mostly based in the northern area of the country and are influenced by tribes of the North such as the Temne, Madingo, and Soso.

Today, the Limba ethnic group makes up the third largest tribe in Sierra Leone, with a total of 592,190 members (8.4%) of the general population, according to the 2015 national census data (Statistics Sierra Leone 2017). The Limba are split between followers of Christianity and Islam depending on their present location, and their interaction with either Christian or Muslim contacts. Despite this fact, a sizeable population of the Limba still practice traditional religion with beliefs in oracles or deities.

The Limba are divided into five dialects. These dialects have been influenced by the tribes that the speakers of each of the five dialects had encountered. The five subgroups include the Sela, Tonko, Safroko, Biriwa, and Wara Wara (Alie 2016). The main secret societies of the Limba men are the Gbangbani, and the Bondo for women. The Limba are mostly peasant farmers and palm wine tappers (a local beverage), and their ceremonies and festivals include initiation ceremonies into either the Gbangbani (for men) and Bondo (for women).

Just as many other ethnic groups who live in rural areas, many Limba use traditional healing methods that utilize herbs and ingredients obtained from the local environment; they also heavily rely on the services of traditional healers. The majority of Limba have embraced Western medicine, with 76 percent of 50 interviewees in the 2020 survey stating that when they are sick—they would exclusively seek out a hospital or clinic to treat their illness. The remaining 24 percent were divided among those that will exclusively consult traditional healers (6%) and those that believe in the power of charms (2%), those relying on prayer to treat illness (14 %), and believers of spiritual healing (2%).

## LOKO

According to a Sierra Leone government survey conducted in 2015, there are approximately 165,000 members of the Loko people in Sierra Leone. In a total population of approximately 7 million people, they represent about 2 percent of all Sierra Leone's population (Statistics Sierra Leone 2015). The major religion adopted by the Loko people is Islam, which, while often mixed with their own ancestral beliefs, is the preferred faith of 70 percent. The second most prolific religion of the Loko is Christianity, which is adopted by 20 percent, with 10 percent still following their own native rites and beliefs (Joshua Project 2020).

Loko men are known for wearing colorful robes and the popular Kufi hat, matching or complementing the colors and patterns of their clothes (Little 2013). The staple crop and core of the Loko cuisine is rice, which is planted on their farms. Other staple crops of the Loko people include cassava, corn, potatoes, peppers, and bananas (Joshua Project 2020). Not many studies are available about the health practices of this group, but it has been reported that quality of health is affected by lack of information on the nature of certain diseases, general distrust of people outside of the tribe, and limited access to treatment centers.

## MANDINGO

The Mandingo people are thought to be the descendants of the Mali Empire; some people think they are the original inhabitants of the ancient city of Djenné-Djenno (Britannica Online Encyclopedia). According to recent statistics, there are currently 160,080 Sierra Leoneans of the Mandingo ethnic group currently living within the borders of the country. This represents approximately 2.3 percent of the nation's total population (Statistics Sierra Leone 2017).

The Mandingo people speak Mandi'nka, which belongs to the Niger-Congo family of languages. Sometimes, because it is the language of the Mandingo/Mandinka people, it is also casually referred to as the Mandingo/Mandinka language. Cultural practices of the Mandingo portray them as patriarchal and thrive on 'clan' culture. Their leadership is by a chief and a group of elders. In the olden days, many of them lived in rural settings alongside trade routes. Arranged marriages are a standard ceremony in this culture.

Mandingo men are known to wear long black gowns, baggy trousers, and a sun shield, while their women, if economically able, wear golden rings in their hair, long gowns, and lappas. Among other articles of traditional Mandingo fashion is the Batik dress, often decorated in vibrant colors and patterns. It is also common for men to wear long flowing robes in similar fashion coupled with a traditional Kufi cap (Little 1949). Peanuts are the main ingredients of the Mandingo people's diet. They also produce millet, corn, sorghum, and rice. Much like other ethnic groups, the health-seeking behaviors of the Mandingo people are influenced by their views on disease and its symptoms.

Fourteen (14) members of this ethnic group were interviewed in our study sample; 40 percent of those respondents believe in the use of clinical medicine while 29 percent claimed to have used the services of traditional healers. The healing power of prayers was also identified as being important to them.

## MENDE

The Mende are mostly located in the southeastern parts of Sierra Leone. According to the National population census of 2015, they are the largest ethnic group, consisting of 2,258,232 people, and accounting for a little over 32 percent of the general population of the country (Statistics Sierra Leone 2017). The traditional religion of the Mende people includes belief in a Creator God, ancestral spirits, and nature deities. Today, many Mende are either Muslims or Christians. The language spoken by this ethnic group is Mende (just as the name of the ethic group itself).

Many Mende in the rural areas are peasant framers who engage in swamp-rice cultivation and fishing. However, many are also cash crop farmers who grow crops such as coffee, and cocoa. The Mende have many different cultural dances among men and women. They grow rice as their staple crop. They also grow yams and cassava. Cocoa, ginger, groundnuts, palm oil, and kernels are used for their cash crops (Little 1949).

This group was represented by 168 respondents in the survey study. Forty-sixty percent of the subsample claimed to believe solely in Western medicine. Believers in traditional medicine accounted for 16 percent of this subsample, while 32 percent confirmed that they could use prayer for combating disease. A little over 5.3 percent indicated belief in either spiritual healing services of sorcerers, or charms.

## SHERBRO

The Sherbro tribe mostly live on an island on the southwestern coast of Sierra Leone. Having absorbed Western customs, the Sherbro have converted to and remained a largely Christian population with other belief systems, having an insignificant impact among them (Anya 1973). The Sherbro speak Sherbro, the language named after their tribe.

For their livelihood, many Sherbro engage in fishing and farming. Their culture is unique for its marriage of African and European values and customs. Dominant clothing for the Sherbro, as with many other ethnic groups of Sierra Leone, is the country's cloth gown, which is often woven into complex patterns of different colors (Wilberforce and McKee 1886). The Sherbro

River plays a great role in the Sherbro diet, as it provides the fish and mangrove rice, which they use for a variety of dishes. Rice is the main crop and is normally served with a variety of stews, sauces, and spices to give extra flavor (Sherbro Foundation 2014).

## SUSU AND YALUNKA

There are approximately 203,779 members of the Susu, and 51,781 Yalunka in Sierra Leone (Statistics Sierra Leone 2017). The Yalunka pray to both, their ancestors and natural spirits, while the Susu have many animistic practices. Today, many members of these ethnic groups are either Muslims or Christians. The Yalunka still practice many of their ancestral rites, such as making sacrifices to their ancestors and to the spirits of nature in exchange for power.

Due to the more isolationist nature of both cultures, combined with the language barrier and a general distrust of outsiders, both Susu and Yalunka tend to resist seeking medical help (Carpenito-Moyet 2006). Among the 11 members of the Susu tribe interviewed, and eight members of the Yalunka tribe, the survey found a high level of trust in Western medicine, with 50 percent of the Susu, and 88 percent of the Yalunka claiming to seek care exclusively in modern clinics. In response to the services of healers, 12 percent of the Yalunka claimed to prefer traditional medicine compared to 36 percent of the Susu, of whom 14 percent also mentioned the effectiveness of prayer for healing purposes.

## TEMNE

The Temne people migrated from the Futa Jallon region of Guinea, who left their original settlements to escape Fulani invasions in the 15th century, and migrated South before settling between the Kolenté and Rokel River area of Sierra Leone (Appiah and Gates 2010). The Temne ethnic group is the second largest ethnic group and consists of 2,220,211 members, (31.6%) of Sierra Leone's population (Statistics Sierra Leone 2017 Census Data). The Temne traditionally believe in a supreme being or a "Creator God." They also believe that witches, both male and female, can make things happen to people, such as have accidents or die. The Temne are Mel-speaking aboriginal people of the Niger-Congo language, and many of them are rice farmers, fishermen, and traders (Ijagbemi 1977). Their culture especially revolves around the Poro society for men, and the Bono society for women. They have elaborate ceremonies associated with crowning ceremonies of local chiefs.

Two hundred and six (206) members of this ethnic group participated in our health-seeking behaviors study. Study data show that there is a significant preference for Western medicine, with 45 percent claiming to seek exclusively the aid of clinics when sick. Traditional beliefs regarding sickness, however, were found to still be expressive among interviewees, with 27 percent exclusively seeking the services of healers versus traditional medicine; 20 percent believe in cure through prayer, 5 percent in using charms, and 3 percent in spiritual healing.

## THE VAI

These individuals originated from Egyptian and Arabic cultures. Also known as the Vei or even the Gallinas, they originated from northwestern Liberia and the boundaries of Sierra Leone, and were named after the local wildfowl, according to early Portuguese writers (Encyclopedia Britannica).

Vai is the smallest ethnic group in Sierra Leone. According to the Sierra Leone 2015 population survey, there are 1,205 members of this group within Sierra Leone. The Via people have been a predominantly Muslim society for centuries. Many of their traditions are centered around the Quran, with a minority of their population declaring themselves Christians. These coexist with the Vai's own traditional beliefs and practices, such as faith in spirits that may do harm upon one person or the entire tribe (Joshua Project). Members of this group practice farming, fishing, including but not limited to weaving and goldsmithing which are their specialties. Among the Vai, traditions are believed that God will manifest himself through spirits and nature that are not lost and keeps them close to their ancestors. The Vai make offerings to deceased family members and other rituals, such as leaving the sacrificial items near their graves as well.

In chapter 1, we explored the relationship between cultural practices and health; in the current chapter, we provided a social context for such practices by briefly describing the ethnic groups in Sierra Leone, some of which are found in other countries within the region. In chapter 3, we will explore specific cultural practices (related to epidemics) while using the 2014–2016 Ebola Outbreak in West Africa as a case study.

## *Chapter 3*

# The Impact of Cultural Practices on Health

## *Case Study of the Ebola Outbreak in Sierra Leone, Liberia, and Guinea*

Mohamed Kanu

In efforts to save lives and improve quality of living for populations across the world, public health and its practitioners grapple with work that characterizes a growing and limitless agenda. This means that when one health challenge is contained or resolved, another is sure to emerge.

During the last few decades, this has been the pattern since the emergence and fight against HIV/AIDS, Bird flu, Ebola, and now the Coronavirus pandemic. Beginning in March 2014 through 2016, the West African region in Sub-Sahara Africa struggled with an Ebola outbreak, which to date remains unprecedented in scope. Among the 17 countries in the subregion, the three countries, Sierra Leone, Liberia, and the Republic of Guinea were the hardest hit. During that time, the resilience of their national health systems, as well as the world's global public health response infrastructure were tested to the core. During the initial stage of the outbreak, the World Health Organization, the world's health governing body, failed to provide the necessary leadership to contain the situation until the virus posed a serious global threat. As infections and the death toll skyrocketed, the international community was morally compelled to respond; subsequently, the outbreak was declared and treated as a public health emergency.

In December 2019 in Wuhan, China, the world witnessed the beginning of another global public health threat—the Coronavirus outbreak (Holshue et al. 2019; WHO 2019). At the time of this writing, the citizens of the world have experienced millions of infections, thousands of fatalities, and grim prospects of yet to be determined long-term health effects. Although Ebola has been largely contained in many parts of Africa where the disease has been dominant, intermittent flare-ups in places such as the Democratic Republic of Congo have remained. This is largely due to local conflicts, which have thwarted the efforts of government and other local and international health agencies or organizations from totally bringing the disease to an end.

The focus of this chapter is an examination of the impact of cultural and religious practices that aided the spread of the Ebola Virus Disease (EVD). Although outbreaks in other countries will be mentioned, more emphasis will be placed on the 2014–2016 Ebola outbreaks in the most affected countries—Sierra Leone, Liberia, and Guinea.

## OTHER HEALTH EMERGENCIES IN WEST AFRICA: SIERRA LEONE, LIBERIA, AND GUINEA

The three countries Sierra Leone, Guinea, and Liberia belong to a region commonly known as the River Mano Basin, with a subregional organization known as the Mano River Union (Steady 2011). At the peak of the Ebola outbreak, Kanu (2014, p. 1) described common characteristics shared by these countries as follows:

"The three West African countries (Guinea, Sierra Leone, and Liberia) that have been most hardly hit by the Ebola outbreak have many things in common, four of which are mentioned here. First, geographically, they share borders that allow the free flow of people from one country to the other with little entry and exit requirement protocols. Second, they have long-standing ethnic relationships that came about when members of the same ethnic group were divided by arbitrary national boundaries created during the colonial period. These ethnic ties, and geographical proximity to one another have also resulted in long-standing trade relations. Business operatives crisscross these national boundaries on daily basis for the purposes of commerce. Third, Liberia and Sierra Leone also experienced brutal civil wars, mostly in the 1980s and 1990s, that ruined their health infrastructure. Although not to the same magnitude, Guinea similarly experienced its own political conflicts that have resulted in the loss of lives and property. Fourth, for a long time, poverty and high illiteracy rates have been affronts to developmental aspirations in all three countries. These geographic, economic, and socio-political commonalities are important characteristics in understanding why the current Ebola outbreak has been so virulent and difficult to contain."

The above commonalities collectively and negatively impacted the already weak health systems in these countries before the Ebola epidemic (Bangura 2021, p. 2). Bangura, a development economist argues that there is a "perceived incapacity of the three [nation]states to domestically finance their development owing to structural rigidities."

Within proximity to one another, many of the Mano River countries, comprising the three original members of Sierra Leone, Liberia, and Guinea, and later Ivory Coast (Steady 2011) tend to "suffer together" during natural calamities (such as floods and landslides) and man-made disasters (such as wars). Between the late 1980s and 2003, Liberia and Sierra Leone jointly experienced some of the most brutal rebel wars in the continent, even by global comparison. The two wars starting in 1989 (Momodu 2016) in Liberia, and 1991 (Beah 2007) in Sierra Leone became so violent and inextricably linked that the orchestrator of the war in Liberia, Mr. Charles Gbangay Taylor, was prosecuted for war crimes by the International Court in the Hague, and is serving time in prison after his conviction for starting the war in his country and supporting the one in Sierra Leone. Similarly, the mastermind of the war in Sierra Leone (Mr. Foday Sankoh) was also convicted, and sentenced to prison, where he later died. Estimates of human fatalities due to these man-made catastrophes are in the thousands.

Between 2013 and 2017, the region again suffered from the double jeopardy of an Ebola disease outbreak and mudslides that killed thousands of citizens in Liberia and Sierra Leone, including health professionals who were already in short supply. Among these calamities, the civil war served as the precursor to other tragedies among which the Ebola epidemic is so far the second most catastrophic. The war led to the loss of thousands of lives, further weakened already fragile health systems, and affected food supplies by temporarily halting agricultural cultivation. As a result, the postwar health systems in these countries remained on "life support." The palpably compromised health systems were incapable of robustly responding to the health problems when Ebola started. During the outbreak, access to and utilization of health services significantly reduced because citizens were afraid to go to health centers for fear of being infected (Govindaraj et al. 2018). Before addressing the cultural factors that hastened the spread of Ebola, it is important to briefly mention how the disease entered the subregion in the first place.

## EARLIER PRESENCE OF EBOLA IN SUB-SAHARAN AFRICA

The March 2014 Ebola outbreak in West Africa was not the first to hit the African continent. Available evidence confirms the presence of the disease in Sub-Saharan Africa that predated the 2014 outbreak. At various times, outbreaks had occurred beginning in Zaire in 1976; in the now Democratic Republic of Congo and Gabon in Central Africa, in Sudan and Uganda in East Africa (Walsh and Johnson 2018). From this evidence, we learned that as many as 34 outbreaks had occurred prior to 2014, although most of them were confined in remote villages, and other highly forested areas (Walsh and Johnson 2018).

Walsh et al. (2018, p. 37) specifically noted that

> Until 2014, the 1976 outbreak, which killed 280 people—88% of those infected, was the deadliest Ebola outbreak in history. Of the 34 outbreaks that had taken place prior to 2014, six outbreaks had each killed more than 100 people, although 17 other outbreaks had killed fewer than 10 people or none at all.

Readers interested in learning more about other outbreaks outside of West Africa can also read the work of Bangura (2021, p. 50) which provides a litany of additional sources on this subject.

## EBOLA IN THE WEST AFRICA SUBREGION—EMPHASIS ON SIERRA LEONE, LIBERIA, AND GUINEA

It was not until 2014 that West Africa experienced its first encounter with the Ebola virus. In varying magnitudes, outbreaks occurred in the West African countries of Sierra Leone, Guinea, Liberia, Mali, Senegal, and Nigeria. Earlier outbreaks which occurred in mostly Central and East Africa took place over an extended period of time, but the West African outbreak happened around the same time—in some cases within weeks of each other: Guinea in December 2013 but was not publicized until March 2014; Sierra Leone in May 2014, and in Lofa County, Liberia, March 30, 2014. By the time the outbreak was contained, the human toll was colossal—upwards of 28,600 infection cases and 11, 325 deaths, according to the Centers for Disease Control and Prevention (CDC 2020).

Ebola in the Mano River Basin was first reported in Guinea in March 2014 (Ansumana et al. 2014). After much speculation, health officials, especially those representing some of the international non-governmental health organizations, such as the WHO and Médecins Sans Frontières (MSF), translated as "Doctors without Borders," confirmed that the first patient of the outbreak (patient zero) was a two-year-old girl in Guinea (Baize, Pannetier, Oestereich et al. 2014). MSF is a French-based international humanitarian organization.

Given Guinea's geographical proximity to Sierra Leone, many believed that the virus would soon reach the shores of Sierra Leone. Indeed, shortly after the disease was officially declared in Guinea, Sierra Leone's first case was also confirmed as a woman who attended a funeral service in Guinea and had returned to Sierra Leone with the virus (Kanu 2014). As Sierra Leoneans remained nervous and uneasy, many more Ebola cases were confirmed by health officials in the weeks that followed. Several of the first cases were diagnosed in the Eastern part of the country in the township of Kenema.

In the West African country of Nigeria, the virus was introduced by an infected sub-regional traveler (from Liberia) who landed in the country's densely populated city of Lagos. The male traveler died a few days later after a few other people were infected (CDC 2014). The disease was quickly contained due to a swift response that was highly applauded. The country's response was characterized by the implementation and adoption of appropriate public health measures including, rapid testing, contact tracing, community engagement of traditional and community leaders, among other efforts. When the outbreak was declared over after 42 days without new infections, the death toll was only in the single digits (see table 3.1 below).

The Republic of Mali had the fifth highest number of cases after Sierra Leone, Liberia, Guinea, and Nigeria. Accounting for only eight confirmed cases and seven deaths, according to WHO data, the introduction of the first case of Ebola infection in this large West African country in October 2014 was traced to the outbreak in Guinea (WHO 2014). With help from WHO and MSF, the government was quickly able to contain the situation without the exponential number of cases reported in other countries.

As in Mali, Ebola found its way into Senegal through a traveler from Guinea. The lone case confirmed to be a man, was treated, recovered fully, and was released, thereby marking the end of the outbreak in that country (WHO 2014).

The EVD had far-reaching impact not only in terms of morbidity and mortality rates. During the outbreak, the then-secretary general of the WHO, Mr.

**Table 3.1 Countries with Widespread Transmission and Other Countries Affected During the Ebola Epidemic**

| *Countries with High Transmissions* | *Total Cases (Suspected, Probable, Confirmed)* | *Lab Confirmed Cases* | *Total Deaths* |
|---|---|---|---|
| Guinea | 3,814 | 3,358 | 2,544 |
| Liberia | 10,678 | 3,163 | 4,810 |
| Sierra Leone | 14,124 | 8,706 | 3,956 |
| Affected Countries | | | |
| Italy | 1 | 1 | 0 |
| Mali | 8 | 7 | 6 |
| Nigeria | 20 | 19 | 8 |
| Senegal | 1 | 1 | 0 |
| Spain | 1 | 1 | 0 |
| United Kingdom | 1 | 1 | 0 |
| United States | 4 | 4 | 1 |
| Total | 28,652 | 15,261 | 11,325 |

*Source*: Centers for Disease Control and Prevention, National Center for Emerging and Zoonotic Infectious Diseases (NCEZID), Division of High-Consequence Pathogens and Pathology (DHCPP), Viral Special Pathogens Branch (VSPB)

Ban Ki-Moon, made a sobering assessment when he said, "The Ebola crisis has evolved into a complex emergency, with significant political, social, economic, humanitarian, and security dimensions. The suffering and spillover effects in the region and beyond demand the attention of the entire world. Ebola matters to us all" (Kanu 2014, p. 3). As noted here, ramifications of the EVD were felt even if indirectly by many countries outside West Africa.

However, in terms of infections and fatalities, a few countries already mentioned borne the brunt of the impact. Of the 17 countries in the region, only three others (Mali, Nigeria, and Senegal), aside from those in the Mano River Basin, reported infections and fatalities. Courtesy of the United States' Centers for Disease Control and Prevention, the table above shows all countries in the Mano River Basin and around the world where infections and fatalities were reported during the infamous 2014 outbreaks.

Although official confirmation of the Ebola outbreak in the affected West African countries constituted a single event in each country, declaring its official end in those countries was a tantalizing process. In three countries, confirmation by the requisite authorities to mark the end of the outbreak was proclaimed more than once as new cases were detected after such announcements. Below is the CDC's summary of how this process occurred in the respective countries.

Liberia was first declared Ebola-free in May 2015. Additional cases were found and treated, and the country was again declared Ebola-free in September 2015. More cases were discovered in November 2015. On January 14, 2016, Liberia again announced it was Ebola-free; however, cases were detected in March and April of 2016, and Liberia made its final declaration on June 1, 2016. After an initial declaration in November 2015, Sierra Leone announced a new case of EVD in January 2016 and declared it was Ebola-free on March 17, 2016. In Guinea, the first end of outbreak declaration was in December 2015, but additional cases were discovered in March and April of 2016. Guinea was finally declared Ebola-free in June 2016 two and a half years after the first case was discovered, the outbreak ended with more than 28,600 cases and 11,325 deaths.

In comparison to the ubiquitous Coronavirus pandemic, the EVD irrespective of its high contagion and lethality, spread into fewer countries. Most of the known and recorded outbreaks had occurred in Africa. By the time of the West African outbreak, most people, including local health professionals and organizations in those countries knew little or nothing about Ebola. Walsh and Johnson (2018, p. 38) attest that "When Ebola was finally confirmed in Guinea in March [2014], there were only three international organizations with significant experience of the disease: the United Nation's World Health Organization (WHO); the US Centers for Disease Control and Prevention (CDC); and the NGO (Médecins Sans Frontieres (MSF)."

## EBOLA AND ITS SYMPTOMS

Today, much more is known about the Ebola virus than when it first emerged in West Africa. For example, it is now common knowledge that this hemorrhagic fever is caused by a virus found in fruit-eating bats. Virologists believe that antelopes and other primates (monkeys, apes, etc.) are infected with the virus when they feed on fruit leftovers from these primates, some of which are consumed by humans as meat (CDC 2014). In the case of West Africa, the viral species of EBOV, Sudan ebolavirus, and Bundibugyo ebolavirus are confirmed as causative agents (Baize, Pannetier, Oestereich et al. 2014). The disease is renowned for its deadliness—as less than half of those infected can recover (Walsh et al. 2018). Others place the fatality rate at greater than 70 percent in some West African countries (Schneider 2020). Many of the signature symptoms associated with the disease include severe fever, muscle pain, fatigue, diarrhea, and vomiting (Schneider 2021).

An infected person's natural immune system deteriorates rapidly, the victim could die within a week of being infected. It may, however, take longer for some people. Quite rapidly the immune system is compromised, partly due to the rapidity with which the virus spreads throughout the body. One writer describes the process thus: "When a person is first infected, the amount of virus in their body is very low, and it is mostly contained within their blood and organs. At this stage, they are unlikely to infect anybody except health workers who come into contact with their blood. As the disease progresses, however, the amount of virus in the body increases exponentially such that there can be more than ten million individual virus particles in one milliliter of blood" (Walsh et al. 2018, p. 35).

Although significant progress has been made in treating victims affected by the Ebola malady with some vaccines and experimental treatments that now prove high efficacy (Schneider 2021), many lingering effects are known to remain among survivors. Some of these post-recovery effects include loss of sight, extreme fatigue, muscular, and joint pain (Schneider 2021) among others.

At the height of the EVD outbreak, finding a cure was not an easy achievement and successive efforts initially went in vain. At that time, infected persons received treatment with what was largely labeled supportive care, convalescent serum, IV fluids, and oral rehydration (Azevedo 2020). Later in 2018–2019; however, a breakthrough with two experimental treatments with REGN-EB3 and mAb-114 brought great relief after others, like ZMAPP were tested in earlier trials. In the 2021 Ebola outbreak in Guinea, the WHO's response was swift when the regional director for Africa, Matshidiso Moeti, announced shortly after the outbreak was confirmed that his organization was sending an initial 11,000 doses of the vaccine and at least 100 experts to help contain the situation.

## THE IMPACT OF TRADITIONAL BELIEFS AND PRACTICES ON THE SPREAD OF THE EVD

Many factors that exacerbated the spread of the Ebola virus in West Africa have been explored by many studies. The focus of this chapter is not to comprehensively explore those factors; rather, it seeks to highlight those that are related to cultural value systems and practices within some of the affected countries.

For millennia, the link between culture and health has been well established. People's cultural values include their health practices which invariably affect their health and general well-being. As so eloquently stated by Skolnik (2021), "Cultural practices, beliefs, customs, and rituals can often increase or mitigate the risk of individuals being exposed to pathogens, which can then affect the transmission patterns of diseases" (Skolnik, p 182).

Before delving into that subject, it is important to differentiate the concepts of illness and disease, from the perspectives of Medical Anthropologists. Michael Winkelman, in his book *Culture and Health* (2009) begins his discussion of the concepts of illness and disease by grouping them into an encompassing category of "Maladies," which he defines as "an umbrella term for unwanted health conditions that encompass many concerns about compromised well-being" (p. 36). Within this umbrella term are the concepts of disease and illness. Regarding the former concept, he writes, "Biomedicine views disease as a biological problem involving abnormality in the body's structure, chemistry, and functions." Illness on the other hand, "refers to a patient's experience of something wrong, a sense of disruption in well-being that may be the results of disease or caused by cultural factors." Michael provides the illustration of how the dichotomy between what doctors view as disease and that which people recognize as illness could lead to miscommunication and affect health outcomes. He cites the example of a health condition known as "lost soul" among the Hmong people, which Western medical doctors perceived to be epilepsy. According to the Hmong, it is possible for a life-soul to be taken from the body of a child by sprits or through other acts (a condition called quab dab peg).

It should not be surprising that biomedical doctors most likely differ about appropriate therapy from local cultural views regarding quab dab peg. Based on the distinction between the two concepts, while illness can be construed as a more subjective cultural connotation, disease is a more objective concept. This means that it is plausible for someone to feel ill and not be diseased, while a diseased person may not yet feel ill until clear symptoms exhibit themselves.

Several cultural practices have been identified as correlates or predictors of health. One factor attributed to the spread of Ebola is Africans' affinity to the extended family values. Africans, especially in Sub-Saharan Africa, are known for their appreciation and acceptance of the extended family values in happier times as well as during times of woes. This includes, but is not limited to caring for sick loved ones, observance of elaborate rituals for the dead, child-naming ceremonies, and other festive events. These are major cultural events that provide rare opportunities for extended families to assemble after long periods of being separated. Sick relatives are often cared for at home and when they die, their bodies are touched. During the epidemic, this show of affection came at a price—sometimes fatal. As described in one publication, "Some African cultures have a traditional solidarity of standing by the sick, which is contrary to the safe care of an Ebola patient" ("West African Cultural Norms/Traditions That May Impact Ebola Transmission": Accessed October 2020).

A second factor associated with the spread of Ebola was the cultural practice of washing human corpses of people who died of the Ebola infection. In their widely acclaimed book about the Ebola outbreak in West Africa, Walsh et al. (2018, p. 35) opined that "When people die of Ebola, their corpse can remain infectious for more than a week and those who touch that corpse to prepare the body for burials can be exposed." Corpse preparers and persons involved in the burial rites may be infected due to exposure to the infected person's blood, vomit, diarrhea, and other bodily fluids. In Guinea, an estimated 60 percent of the Ebola cases in 2014 were attributed to burial-related practices (Alexander et al. 2015).

Also, during the initial stages of the outbreak, governments (as reported in Sierra Leone) tried to adopt rigid public health measures by encouraging "stay in place" practices, which is a concept meant to restrict the movement of people from place to place to reduce rapid disease spread. Rather than complying, some families encouraged or even facilitated movement of potentially infected family members to other locations to avoid stigma and/or government-imposed quarantine. This practice was frequently done during the night to avoid being detected by authorities. (interview with community member in Sierra Leone, December 2019)

The spread of Ebola in West Africa was also intensified by people's belief in and use of traditional medicines, originally believed to cure Ebola-infected persons. At the beginning of the outbreak, treatment was unavailable, and hospitals and other health facilities only provided supportive care (stabilizing the patient with adequate fluids and supplements rather than actual treatment medication). At this time, many people used any help they could get. In some communities, infected patients stayed away from other health care facilities, which increased the chances of spreading the infection to other family and community members.

Especially during the early stages of the outbreak, even supportive care was limited, and basic physical structures such as isolation centers were in short supply. In the absence of adequate pharmaceutical supplies in cultures, where people have heavily relied on traditional medicine for ages, many could not be prevented from the extensive use of these remedies. Some scholars have aptly described this situation by saying that, in addition to traditional West African healers having used herbal remedies for a long time, the West African people also trust these treatments and find them to be less expensive in comparison to imported medication (James, Wardle, et al. 2018; Skolnik 2021).

While many conspiracy theories are bogus, some are based on peoples' real experiences which then shape part of their beliefs within communities. For many years, suspicion and conspiracy theories against biomedicine and some of its practitioners have been largely discussed in Western cultures. The treatment of prisoners by Nazi Germany doctors when unsuspecting prisoners served as study participants without consent, and African Americans in the United States during the infamous Tuskegee Syphilis Study are towering examples of medical malpractice (Smith and Davis 2013). To date, many believe that the difficulty faced by medical practitioners in recruiting minorities into clinical studies is partially attributed to fear of abuse of minority groups. These examples are not limited to Western experience alone, but have had far-reaching impact on African and other countries. During the Ebola pandemic, resistance to Western medical practitioners was encountered within some affected countries.

Several reasons have been advanced to explain the West African resistance to treatment by Western health professionals. They range from accusations of disruption of African-style burial practices by Western medical practices (James, Wardle, et al. 2018), allegations of ineffectiveness of biomedical treatments, accusations of Western practitioners of introducing the virus to Africans for research purposes, and claims of a campaign to harvest organs from Ebola victims (Gassel 2014). These beliefs and assertions, largely based on cultural differences, significantly thwarted biomedical efforts in quickly prohibiting the spread in a timely manner. In the Republic of Liberia, locals were reported to hide relatives infected with Ebola from health professionals and buried them secretly when they died (Nyenswah, Kateh 2016). At the time, even unconfirmed rumors about alleged infection status could subject victims and their families to ostracization, and shunned treatment by other community members (Skolnik 2021).

## Empirical Data on Ebola-Related Cultural Perceptions among Some Ethnic Groups in West Africa

Understanding local perceptions about the cause and spread of infectious diseases, especially in underdeveloped nations is critical for health professionals. Quite often, factors such as high levels of illiteracy rates, poverty, inaccessibility to health information, and cultural practices, have made health intervention programs more difficult to implement. To address perceptions about the spread of infectious diseases, it is important to comprehend what people in affected communities believe about disease causation. Anthropologists have long explored the subject of disease causation in non-Western societies. Foster (1998) described causes of disease in these societies according to two typologies.

The first is what he named the Personalistic medical system, where disease is believed to occur "due to the active, purposeful intervention of an agent, who may be human (a ghost, an ancestor, an evil spirit), or supernatural (a deity or other very powerful being)." The belief here, he writes, is that "the sick person literally is a victim, the object of aggression or punishment directed specifically against him, for reasons that concern him alone" (p. 112). It is conceivable that a deceased parent ancestor, in retaliation for neglectful behavior of a surviving child for such disloyal or ungrateful acts (i.e., non-offering of prayers by the grave side), may inflict punishment on that child. This author remembers hearing stories like this while growing up in Sierra Leone.

Forster (1998) also describes the second medical system as the Naturalistic medical system in which disease causation is attributed to a disequilibrium in the substances within the human body. Rather than resulting from the "machinations of an angry being," illness is caused by "natural forces or conditions as cold, heat, winds, dampness" (p. 112). According to this typology, the human anatomy consists of hot and cold substances that must always be at a level of equilibrium, any imbalance will cause illness.

The contrast to the two systems described in the preceding paragraphs is the biomedical model prevalent in Western medical systems where disease is caused by pathogens. In this context, diseases are caused by germs such as bacteria and viruses. As observed by Brown, Inhorn and Smith (Brown et al. 1996, p. 186), "for the practitioner of biomedicine, disease is the expression of pathology alone." As to be expected, just as diseases are perceived to be caused by different agents, so are the corresponding systems of diagnosis and techniques of correct therapies. Even the most universal and rigorously researched biomedical treatment regimens of today will be of little use if the affected patients hold doubtful views about the efficacy of these treatments.

Many studies have been conducted during and after the end of Ebola in West Africa to assess knowledge levels about the cause and transmission of the disease, and it is accurate to say that post-Ebola awareness about the cause and transmission of the disease in many communities, is higher compared to pre-outbreak levels. Four years after the scourge came to an end, the study described in earlier sections of this book was conducted to assess some of the lingering beliefs associated with Ebola. The following paragraphs provide a summary of the study findings as they relate to cultural perceptions and belief systems. Five hundred (500) respondents drawn from mostly urban and peri-urban settlements in Sierra Leone were asked questions ranging from cultural beliefs and practices that potentially exposed people to the Ebola infection, causes of Ebola, loss of close and distant relatives to Ebola, as well as views about how Ebola survivors should be perceived/treated by community members.

As presented earlier in the chapter, one of the factors responsible for the widespread of Ebola during the epidemic was seeking treatment from traditional healers, especially during the early period of the outbreak. Two general (non-Ebola related) questions were asked to assess belief in the power of traditional healing practices and the frequency of use of those services during the past 12 months. In response to the first question, 41 percent acquiesced to their belief in the healing power of traditional medicine; however, a greater percentage of respondents (60.9%) had used the services at one time or another during the past 12 months.

In terms of knowledge about the cause of Ebola, 84.3 percent correctly identified the cause of the illness as a virus, while the remainder of the respondents thought the disease was caused by factors such as infected blood, bad air, curse, evil spirits, and "other" factors. Although, the respondents with incorrect knowledge are in the minority, they represent 16 percent of the study sample, which is significant since many of them reside in peri-urban or urban communities where health information is more readily available than for dwellers in more rural settings. It is not certain whether this is due to genuine lack of knowledge, or inability to recall correct information after the end of the outbreak.

Although some fatalities that occurred during the epidemic were not directly related to Ebola (due to less utilization of hospital services during the epidemic), many deaths were directly Ebola-related. In the current study, respondents reported to have lost friends, community, and/or immediate family members. According to study data, 38.3 percent of respondents repoted that they lost friends due to Ebola, approximately 55 percent lost community members, and 30.2 percent lost an immediate family member. Perceptions about type of treatment to be meted out to Ebola survivors were mixed. Sixteen-nine percent (69%) agreed or strongly agreed that survivors must not be ostracized to prevent reinfection and/or stigma; Twenty-four percent (24%); however, thought this was necessary. The remainder of respondents expressed no opinion.

As previously mentioned, one critical practice considered to be a "super spreader" of Ebola infection was the practice of washing deceased persons before burial. In the survey, the question was asked whether respondents agreed that this practice was an important cultural or religious attribute that must be continued; 37.3 percent agreed, and 55 percent strongly agreed that the practice must be maintained. Only 4.72 percent favored the discontinuation of the practice while 2.4 percent expressed no opinion. Ironically, most of the respondents believed that the practice of washing bodies constituted a high risk of infection to its practitioners. When asked if this traditional practice would put handlers at greater risk of contracting Ebola, 93.6 percent of respondents answered in the affirmative. The two contrasting findings show a conflict between strongly held beliefs on the one hand, and serious health risks associated with those beliefs on the other. Such empirical findings provide an opportunity for public health professionals to design not only safe health intervention programs, but ones that are also culturally sensitive.

## NON-CULTURAL FACTORS THAT AIDED THE SPREAD OF EBOLA

The reasons for the spread of Ebola are not limited to cultural factors alone. A litany of other reasons mentioned in the extant literature include an initial lackluster response by the WHO, the large and unprecedented scale of the outbreak, unpreparedness of affected countries to respond robustly (Kanu 2014), myths about the cause of the outbreak, deliberate misinformation or based on political partisanship machinations, weak health systems (CDC 2019), and poor coordination of response efforts by affected governments, among other factors.

Weak health systems constituted a limited capacity to robustly respond to the Ebola outbreak, especially during the early stages. In varying degrees of limitations, health systems in many West African countries were grossly understaffed and contained hundreds of poorly trained personnel, inadequately funded (Worthington 2014) and often characterized by corruption. At the beginning of the outbreak, very little accurate information about the EVD was available. To add to the confusion, many locals disseminated fabrications that governments were peddling information about the outbreak to receive donor funds; others simply disbelieved and maintained that no such disease existed.

As many infectious disease experts have predicted, the threat of infectious disease is going to be an omnipresence in many communities for the foreseeable future. Since 2016 when the Ebola outbreak was declared over in West Africa, no other flares of the disease had been reported elsewhere within the region until recently, in the middle of February 2021, when a new outbreak was announced by the Government of the Republic of Guinea in a region called Nzerekore. Early in the month of March, the outbreak left 18 people sick, and another nine people dead (Kupferschmidt 2021). This time, the immediate response of the West African region, as well as that of the WHO is commendable. In all three countries, the response systems set in place during the 2014 outbreaks were activated and surveillance processes were heightened. Similarly, the WHO, in addition to sending experts to help trace and isolate infected persons through contact tracing, also flew a plane in with vaccines to inoculate many local residents. To date, the cases of new infections have not skyrocketed as was the case in 2013–2014, and that should be credited to the coordinated actions of health officials in these countries and the collaboration with WHO, MSF, International Organization for Migration, and many other agencies.

During the 2014 outbreak, it was confirmed that males who previously tested positive for the disease could carry the virus in their semen for longer periods after they previously appeared to be free of the disease. Diallo et al. (2016) confirmed that the virus could be in the semen for a little over 500 days. The re-emergence of the virus in Guinea has taken this confirmation to another level when researchers alleged that the index case or patient zero in Guinea, confirmed to be a 51-year-old nurse (thought to be cured) had the virus which lay dormant for about five years. The virus was found in the blood of her husband. Writing about this sad state of affairs, Branswell (2021, p. 1), describes the study analysis that led to the recent confirmation as follows: "The analysis suggests that a survivor of the historic Ebola outbreak continued harboring the virus at least five years after being infected, eventually transmitting it to someone."

The long latency period of the Ebola virus could pose serious cultural implications for marriage relationships. In these countries and many others in the region, polygamy is widely practiced and a virus that lodges in the male's seminal fluid for many years only to become infectious again, poses a high risk of infection for his wives and anyone else in the love triangle. This is in addition to the stigmatization of those who survived the dreaded disease. As observed by an infectious disease doctor, the finding raises serious questions about further stigmatizing survivors. A cultural implication is the future survival of marriages if married couples can establish that partners, especially males can carry the virus in their seminal fluids for a long time, with the possibility of reinfection for the partner. Important questions can be raised about this situation, such as how will spouses react to situations when their partners survive the disease but feared to be carrying the virus? Will marriages be affected because of this?

Many of the affected countries were unprepared at the time of the outbreak. Health systems were under-resourced in personnel, equipment, funding, as well as supplies. As noted by Adeyi (2018, p. xi), "With the end of that Ebola outbreak, the World Bank's engagement in Guinea, Liberia, and Sierra Leone, shifted from a response effort toward a focus on rebuilding and strengthening the very foundations of health systems that were already weak prior to the crisis." Alongside the operation of weak health systems that largely failed to provide routine health services to citizens, the EVD outbreak turned out to be the biggest outbreak in recorded history. The scale of the epidemic (with thousands of lab-confirmed infections and upwards of 11,000 deaths) produced ripple effects that impacted the social, political, and economic facets of the affected nations.

Some valuable time was lost in planning the technical response during the beginning of the epidemic. Because of its experience and global leadership credentials, the WHO was looked upon for guidance by affected countries. A combination of factors impacted its initial performance in responding to the crisis. According to Walsh et al. (2018), the response was initially relaxed because some WHO officials with Ebola experience from Central Africa thought that the West African outbreak was going to be confined to a limited geographical area, as previously seen elsewhere in other parts of Africa. MSF saw this differently due to the rapid pace in which infected and healthy people were interacting.

Furthermore, the WHO was also experiencing budgetary cuts that affected the recruitment of quality and quantity of staff members. As reported by one US newspaper, a top US government official described the WHO Africa office at the time as "A place where politics often trumps substance and where key appointees often are not the cream of the crop" (Walsh et al. 2018, p. 41). It is undeniable that political considerations and diminishing global budgets affected the initial response efforts against the Ebola epidemic by the WHO, who many national governments heavily rely on for guidance during global health crises.

## *Chapter 4*

# Integrating Cultural and Behavioral Adaptations in Disease Prevention

Mohamed Kanu

Many factors presented in chapter 3 exacerbated the spread of Ebola in the same way as many behavioral lifestyles have impacted other disease outbreaks (e.g., cholera), and other health emergencies such as mudslides and flooding. This chapter will discuss national efforts (in Sierra Leone and other Ebola-affected countries) at standardizing the modus operandi of non-Western traditional healers and other cultural practice models developed by or recommended by reputable organizations such as the World Health Organization, and others. Behavioral change theories/models associated with health-related cultural practices are also examined.

### DEFINITION OF TRADITIONAL AND COMPLEMENTARY MEDICINE

Traditional and complementary medicine (T&CM) is defined as the combined use of different health products and practices which are unassociated with the conventional or dominant health care system and medical profession (WHO 2002). Although the concepts of traditional medicine and complementary medicine are presented as inseparable in most discussions, the WHO points out the distinction between the two. Traditional medicine implies "a comprehensive term used to refer both to traditional medical systems such as traditional Chinese medicine, Indian ayurveda, and Arabic unani medicine, and to various forms of indigenous medicine" (p. 1). The ingredients used in the development of these remedies may be obtained from the local community or brought from elsewhere. The treatment regimen may, or may not, include the use of medication. When medication is required in the treatment, substances obtained from herbs, animal parts or other minerals may be used.

At times, no medication is directly used such as in circumstances when remedies as acupuncture and spiritual healings are used. (WHO 2002).

## COMPLEMENTARY MEDICINE

In some countries, the practice of traditional medicine is not fully standardized. In developed countries, science-based medicine, otherwise known as allopathic medicine, characterizes the dominant health system. Complementary medicine refers to a health care provision found in countries where allopathic medicine is predominant but traditional medicine has not been incorporated into the national health system (WHO 2002). Such a system is also referred to as alternative or non-conventional medicine. In many Western countries as the United States of America, acupuncture (an example of alternative medicine) has gained some traction in recent years; however, it is still not extensively practiced or largely integrated into the dominant health system.

## ARGUMENTS IN FAVOR OF TRADITIONAL MEDICINE

The World Health Organization provides some distinction between traditional medicine and complementary alternative medicine. In their use of the terms, "traditional medicine" is used when referring to regions such as Africa, Latin America, Southeast Asia, and/or the Western Pacific, whereas "complementary and alternative medicine" is used when reference is made to Europe and/or North America (and Australia) (WHO 2005, p. 1). When referring in a general sense to these regions, the comprehensive TM/CAM is used.

While the use of traditional medicine is growing in developing countries, complementary and alternative medicine (CAM) is known to be increasing in developed nations. Data from the WHO indicate that up to 80 percent of the population use traditional medicine. The pervasive use in these lower income countries has occurred due to various reasons, some of which are presented in the following paragraphs.

First, it is known to be affordable for many impoverished families (WHO 2002). It is common knowledge that many individuals in impoverished nations around the world live on the equivalent of less than one dollar a day. For people in this income bracket, traditional medicine, often without charges, such as doctor consultation fees, expensive necessary lab tests, and sometimes occupancy fees incurred during extended stays in hospitals, is not only appealing but the only thing they can afford.

A second reason for the popularity of traditional medicine is people's cultural affinity to it. According to the WHO, populations in Asia and Latin

America continue to "use TM as a result of historical circumstances and cultural beliefs. In China, their use of traditional medicine account for 40 percent of healthcare" (WHO, p. 1). For millennia, communities across the world have been accustomed to the use of these remedies. Within some ethnic groups in Africa (e.g. the Temnes of Sierra Leone), knowledge about the potency of traditional medicine has been handed down from generation to generation. The oldest surviving members of a family who are custodian of such knowledge pass on the wisdom to younger members of the same family or of other households within the community.

The ever presence of herbal remedies within communities across developing countries has made traditional medicine an indispensable attribute of their existence. In Africa and Southeast Asia, for example, the distribution of health facilities is often without regard to population density (Merson et al. 2012). In some of these countries, the majority of the population work and live in rural areas. Ironically, these are the areas with fewer health facilities and medical supplies. In this scenario of increasing population growth against insufficient health facilities, local herbal remedies will most likely fill the void.

Associated with the above factor is the low number of allopathic health personnel in developing countries as a whole. Generally, the health professional to population ratio is lopsided. During the Ebola outbreak in 2014, Sierra Leone and Liberia had a ratio of about two doctors to every 100,000 people in their respective countries (Worthington 2014). This problem is worst in rural areas because many health workers prefer to settle and work in urban communities. This uneven distribution of health services providers leaves residents in rural and peri-urban communities, having to heavily rely on traditional remedies.

As Africans witnessed during the Ebola epidemic, many people in affected countries were suspicious of biomedicine, which also pushed them to use traditional medicine as the natural alternative. Although many people prefer traditional over biomedicine because it is less expensive, others dislike biomedicine because of Western clinical personnel suspected of dubious and ulterior motives. At times, the suspicion held against Western practitioners is extended to the therapies they provide to local beneficiaries.

Locals have faith in the therapies provided for them by local healers. When there are no infectious disease emergencies such as Ebola, cholera, and others, and governments clamp down on local practitioners in order to prevent disease spread, the demand for the services of local health practitioners is generally high. From discussions in previous chapters, there is evidence that in low-income countries citizens in rural and urban communities utilize a medley of formal and informal, traditional and biomedical, spiritual and many "self-certified" healthcare providers. The motivation for the combined sources of care is "influenced by a number of factors, including supply side factors (proximity and cost), previous experiences of care, disease specific factors . . . and personal and community beliefs about the appropriateness of different strategies" (Idris et al. 2020, p. 1).

## LEGITIMACY OF TRADITIONAL MEDICINE WITHIN EBOLA-AFFECTED COUNTRIES

Establishing regulatory policies and processes is an important first step in the practice of traditional medicine in countries where record keeping is generally poor. That is the situation in many Sub-Saharan African countries. Regulations that exist in theory only will do little to improve healthcare, unless there are stiff sanctions for the different health practitioners within a system.

In a study conducted by the World Health Organization in 1992, many countries around the world were found to have some form of supervision over traditional healers. West African countries affected by the Ebola outbreak similarly had some regulatory or structural systems related to the practice of traditional medicine. This is important because these traditional healers were found to have sometimes unknowingly helped to spread the Ebola virus when they treated Ebola victims (Hewlett et al. 2003). In Guinea, the country was reported to have official legislative and regulatory provisions that govern the practice of TM. Practitioners have a licensing process and interdepartmental councils related to the practice of traditional medicine (WHO 1992).

As far back as 1966, Sierra Leone had recognized the value of traditional medicine through the Medical and Dental Surgeons Act by not expressly forbidding the practice of customary treatments. The more recent Traditional Medicines Act of 1996 attempts to regulate the practice of traditional medicine within the county, although many will argue that it needs more rigid enforcement. To prevent Ebola transmission through contact with traditional healers, the government instituted fiscal sanctions including potential incarceration for non-compliant traditional healers, who were mandated to form an association with formal membership.

As recounted by Pa Komrabai, traditional healers were required to send all persons seeking treatment to hospitals first, then bring a clearance to traditional healers, proving they had been seen in a hospital before traditional healers attend to them (Kassaye 2015). Today, the Traditional Healers Association serves as an umbrella organization through which the government can exercise some oversight of local healers.

The Republic of Liberia sanctions the practice of traditional medicine as established in its legislative and regulatory processes. As reported in the literature, "There is a registry of traditional health practitioners, and local and national councils for traditional medicine. Local officials are allowed to authorize the practice of traditional medicine in their administrative and/or health subdivisions, and some traditional medicine practitioners are involved in Liberia's primary health care programme" (WHO 1992, p. 20).

In Mali, it is reported that greater than 70 percent of the population uses traditional medicine and with such numbers, prohibition of the practice by authorities would have been impossible. In 1973, the Department of Traditional Medicine and the National Research Institute of Medicine and Traditional Medicine were created and local practitioners, who operate as herbalists and therapists are members. These local practitioners are issued membership cards perceived to be useful for regulatory purposes. The establishment of these regulatory institutions was meant "to demonstrate the value of traditional medicine resources through scientific research and to differentiate the roles of herbalists from those of other traditional medicine practitioners, which included defining their respective status, regulations, and code of ethics" (p. 22).

The Federal Republic of Nigeria, the most populous nation in Africa has recognized the practice of traditional medicine for a long time. Earlier efforts to regulate the practice have been reported; however, they were not formalized until 1966, following research work done by the University of Ibadan on the medicinal value of local herbs. In the 1980s, policies allowed the accreditation and registration of traditional medicine practitioners (WHO 1992). During the same decade, the Federal Ministry of Health supported the establishment of the National Investigative Committee on Traditional and Alternative Medicine with broad oversight of these practitioners. Given Nigeria's population, it is conceivable why the government had moved in earlier years to institute some form of standardization for the practice of traditional healing. Even with these efforts to regulate the practice of traditional medicine, many problems remain. Sub-Saharan Africa has some of the world's highest illiteracy rates and trying to upgrade anything that requires reading would be a demanding undertaking. Some of the challenges associated with traditional medicine are briefly examined in the next paragraphs.

## CHALLENGES ASSOCIATED WITH THE USE OF TRADITIONAL MEDICINE

Practice protocols between allopathic and traditional medicine are and will remain very distinct. While the former relies on tested and proven standards of operation, the latter remains largely untested, and its processes and procedures are less streamlined. Biomedical practice models are standardized across the globe. Knowledge acquisition and its transfer from person to person follow stipulated criteria, such as years of schooling which require theoretical and practical competence, passing exams, and completing many years of apprenticeship.

In spite of the popularity of traditional medicine in many parts of the world, its use is also associated with serious challenges. Many of its practitioners are not formally trained and the efficacy of some of the treatments is sometimes questionable. According to the World Health Organization, "In many parts of the world, policymakers, health professionals, and the public are wrestling with questions about the safety, efficacy, quality, availability, preservation and further development of this type of health care" (WHO 2002, p. 1). This is particularly critical during health emergencies when alternative health services may be in short supply or the general public may reduce consumption of services if the health emergency is associated with the spread of infectious diseases.

Based on concerns expressed about the safety of TM, necessary efforts must be undertaken to standardize some of the paraphernalia associated with its practice to improve this critical component of the health industry. This is critically important because traditional medicine is delivered within social-cultural contexts and the two are inseparable. Even when the medicine may be desirable, the socio-environmental context within which it is delivered may be compromised, and that part of it may be improved. The next section highlights some practice and policy-related efforts that are necessary to achieve this objective.

## THE ARGUMENT FOR REFINING HEALTH-RELATED CULTURAL PRACTICES AND REGULATING AND STANDARDIZING TRADITIONAL MEDICINE

Traditional medicine is the nucleus of healthcare for many rural and peri-urban residents in many developing countries. As one author noted, "People generally go to a provider who is from their community, speaks their language, is known to them, and treats them with respect, rather than an outsider who may be disrespectful." He goes further to say that, "people around the world tend to treat illness at home and then go to the local healer" (Skolnik 2021, p. 171). Therefore, in spite of its noted limitations, healers have earned the trust of those they serve. In addition to the trust, dissatisfaction with Western biomedicine (James et al. 2018), which is supposed to be the alternative, leaves traditional medicine the only option available to multitudes of people who desperately need care. Because of the appealing attributes of TM to both providers and beneficiaries, it is hard to imagine that its practice will ever be abandoned. Rather than advocating abandonment, efforts toward improvement are more plausible and must be vigorously pursued.

As discussed earlier in this chapter, a World Health Organization study (2002) provided a status report about countries with or without some form of supervisory systems over the practice of traditional medicine. The study documented countries with legislative provisions and training programs for practitioners of TM. Consistent with that review, this chapter offers two broad approaches toward improvements in TM. These approaches relate to policies and practitioners, and general health-related behavioral lifestyles.

The first approach relates to policy and practitioner-related factors. It focuses on improving the full repertoire of treatment processes and procedures used by traditional healers through policies that guide those practices. Stated differently, the emphasis of this approach must be to upgrade standards of practice used by traditional practitioners through regulatory provisions, training, and adoption of vetted practices. For example, during the Ebola outbreak, traditional healers in Sierra Leone were prohibited by law from treating locals, until the latter produced evidence showing that they had first reported and were screened in a hospital. Relating to cultural practices, the World Health Organization (WHO 2014) developed and introduced the culturally sensitive 12-step Safe and Dignified Burial protocol. This protocol, later used in the affected countries, helped to prevent the spread of infections because it was carefully vetted and culturally sensitive to burial practices of indigenous populations.

The second approach relates to behavioral lifestyle changes by members of the general public. This approach must target the societal behavioral lifestyle through the use of scientifically proven behavioral science theories in health intervention programs.

The use of traditional healing is an integral part of culture in many developing countries. For years to come, allopathic medicine will coexist with traditional medicine. The two need not be integrated, but the latter can learn a lot from the more established standards of the former.

Improved training for traditional healers is critical for enhancing health outcomes among users of traditional medicine. Due to the lack of training, many traditional healers are less likely to pay serious attention to safety issues, such as dispensation or quantity of the therapies they recommend. For example, it is a known fact that in native treatment, healers instruct "patients" to drink local concoctions as much as they can drink without regard to overdose. Another example involves fractures where healers use herbs for healing within the first few minutes of an occurrence of the fracture, rather than keeping the fractured limbs in place for proper alignment. Practitioners of this type should be trained in first aid processes to improve the prognosis of a patient with fractured limbs, which is a common occurrence in many rural settings, many of which have no biomedical doctors.

An area of improvement for traditional medicine is policy requirements regarding proof of efficacy of some therapies. For example, requiring information labeling about ingredients used by healers in preparing their remedies is an important first step. As James and his colleagues have noted, traditional medicine is used in Africa with assurances of effectiveness even when there is no scientific proof of its efficacy (James et al. 2019). Rather than undergoing training and displaying certificates of training, healers often claim to have knowledge passed on to them by older family members or others in their communities. For example, one traditional healer boasted by saying, "I inherited the skills and knowledge to be a traditional healer from my grandfather," I studied the plants and I know which ones cure, and I was very successful. People saw my abilities to cure things—especially when people came suffering from witch-gun (witchcraft). So, they made me chief traditional healer" (Kassaye 2015, p. 5). The truth is that many of these practitioners have not undergone training, and clients who use their services do so at their own risk. Instituting required training programs will help improve services and save lives.

Closely related to the issue of efficacy of traditional therapies is that of safety concerns. Safety is simply the most critical aspect of TM where regulatory policies can make a significant impact. Unsafe use of local therapies can occur when healers pay no heed or are not informed about dosage limits, giving false assurances to patients by claiming knowledge to heal ailments which they have no ability to treat, using crude equipment that are inappropriate and unsterilized. Government policies can institute training and supervisory regulations to address these and many other safety-related issues. Along with training requirements, there must be mandatory regulations for registration with local authorities within the jurisdiction of practice.

At times cultural practices have implications for health. The infamous practice of female circumcision is a notable example. This practice is common in many West African countries, and for many years testimonies provided by initiates depict the use of crude instruments that can be better sanitized. As this practice remains hard to eliminate, additional focus should be placed on training its practitioners to use better equipment and safer procedures. Regulatory sanctions must be serious to include strict fines and/or incarceration which are commensurate with the gravity of the crime.

During the Ebola epidemic, traditional burial practices represented one mode of viral transmission at the beginning of the outbreak. Family members who lost loved ones to Ebola in some of the affected countries performed traditional burials as a show of affection to the deceased (Hewlett et al. 2003). Transmission of the virus was exacerbated by this practice until the introduction of the safe burial protocol by the WHO. This was a recognition of traditional preferences, such as praying for the body before burial while avoiding direct contact with the body. This compromise assured cultural sensitivity while upholding the tenets of good public health practice. Many countries in West Africa have made significant efforts to improve the combined use of traditional medicine along with that of biomedicine. Governments have implemented more regulatory processes that guide the practice of traditional medicine; they have adopted scientifically safer methods of dealing with tenuous situations involving health-related cultural practices and risk of infection (e.g., safe Ebola victims' burials), and guidelines on how to engage communities to enhance social mobilizations among the citizenry during health emergencies.

In many developing countries, where there is coexistence of what some have termed as medical pluralism, which is the combined use of conventional and TM (James et al. 2019), the need to improve the latter with its inherent problems already discussed, cannot be overemphasized. Improving the ubiquitous traditional healing practices requires a careful examination of policies governing the practice of TM, procedures and processes that characterize traditional healing, and behavioral lifestyles (impacted by cultural practices) of the consumers of these services. Policies must include those in the private and public domains with more emphasis on the latter because they are backed by government for enforcement purposes. Due to the inextricable link between cultural practices and behavioral lifestyles, the next section will examine how select behavioral change theories may be used to improve health outcomes.

## CULTURE, BEHAVIORAL LIFESTYLES AND BEHAVIORAL CHANGE THEORIES AND MODELS

A significant connection to be realized is that health behaviors are related to culture. Preventing illness and improving health; therefore, requires a comprehensive and holistic approach to address the determinants of health that include access to health services, genetic factors, socio-economic and environmental factors, and behavioral factors (Turnock 2009). For developing countries, placing premium on prevention through interventions targeting health behaviors is extremely critical as these countries already lack well-funded, sophisticated, and improved health systems that will treat people after they become ill.

As low-income countries such as those in West Africa continue to deal with meager financial budgets for health sectors spending, it is not surprising that many health care providers and users of health services combine indigenous practices with allopathic or Western biomedicine. With this combination, even more lives will be saved if additional emphasis is placed on prevention by focusing particularly on improving behavioral lifestyles. Risk factors responsible for some of the highest causes of premature deaths are related to behavioral lifestyles in many countries (Turnock 2009).

Behaviors that are inimical to human health are many; they include, but are not limited to, poor diets, substance abuse (such as alcohol consumption and smoking), unsafe sex, sedentary lifestyles or not performing adequate physical activity, and reckless or unsafe driving. In public health terminology, all these behaviors are described as modifiable factors because people can take actions or do something to improve them. It is for that reason that deaths caused by any of these behaviors are often regarded as preventable mortality. When people make conscious efforts to improve behavioral lifestyles, morbidity rates, mortality, and general quality of life may be improved. As good as this may sound, changing unhealthy behaviors and adopting healthy ones is not simple for many people, old and young alike. The remainder of this chapter will explore a few behavioral science theories and models that focus on improving behavioral lifestyles.

According to Glanz et al. (1997), a theory is "a set of interrelated concepts, definitions, and propositions that presents a systemic view of events or situations by specifying relations among variables in order to explain and predict the events or situations" (p. 21). The authors state further that the purpose of theories and models is to "explain behavior and suggest ways to achieve behavioral change" (p. 23).

One of the most referenced among the health behavior theories is the Health Belief Model, developed by psychologists within the United States Public Health Service in the 1950s (Hochbaum 1958). The model seeks to explain why people fail to take actions that may prevent or ameliorate the impact of diseases or other health conditions that may afflict them. The foundation of the theory is based on a desire to understand why people were reluctant or refused to be tested for tuberculosis through the use of x-rays (Hochbaum 1958). The theory is based on the idea that people will act to prevent a disease or health condition only if they believe in any of the following factors (Strecher and Rosenstock 1997):

- They are susceptible or could get the illness.
- The disease could result in severe consequences if they get it.
- There are benefits associated with preventing the illness.
- The potential health benefits, resulting from taking early action, are worth the barriers to be faced in doing so.

This means that unless people believe in one or more of the conditions listed above, they are less likely to do anything to prevent or take immediate actions to stop the illness. In the case of the TB (Tuberculosis) x-ray study, more people who believed that they could develop TB allowed themselves to be screened than those who did not. This is analogous to many of the behaviors witnessed across communities today, that people who have a false sense of security toward a particular illness are less inclined to take necessary preventive measures.

## THE STAGES OF CHANGE OR TRANSTHEORETICAL MODEL

The Stages of Change Model explains the human behavioral change process as a series of steps along a continuum rather than a single event. Prochaska et al. (1997) explain that people go through six (6) steps in the behavioral change process as listed below:

Precontemplation—a stage where the individual has no plan of making a change in behavior in the near future, usually estimated to be within the next 6 months.

Contemplation—the individual is considering a change within the next 6 months but no final decision has yet been made.

Preparation—when change is imminent or will occur within a month, when some readiness steps may have been taken during the past months.

Action—at this stage, the individual has taken some observable actions during the past six months related to the intended behavioral change.

Maintenance—the person at this stage is able to maintain the behavior and usually capable of preventing or avoiding a relapse.

Termination—when the person is 100 percent confident about having adopted the new behavior and a relapse is unlikely.

The main emphasis of this model is that human behavioral change is not an automatic process; it entails a series of steps that occur over time. In addition to understanding that critical fact, the model provides guidance for implementers of intervention programs to understand the essence of matching intervention activities, in accordance with the stage of change of program beneficiaries. For example, a smoking cessation program for smokers in the precontemplation stage must design activities that program participants have not considered quitting smoking, which means the earliest activity must focus on demonstrating the merits of cessation before other activities are planned along the continuum. Program activities must reflect the stage of change for program participants; otherwise, they will be less successful.

## THE SOCIAL ECOLOGICAL MODEL

It has been established that multiple factors, both internal and external to the individual, determine a person's health. The Social Ecological Model recognizes that behaviors are influenced by environmental factors in the same way as individuals can impact the environment they live in (Hayden 2019). This symbiotic relationship is depicted in the proverbial saying that people are products of their environments. Imbedded in the ecological framework is the idea that influence on health behaviors span a continuum of five levels. People's behaviors and health are impacted by these five levels of factors that include intrapersonal factors (such as knowledge, beliefs, attitudes), interpersonal factors (such as social support), institutional or organizational factors, community, and policy level factors. It must be understood that health interventions aimed at creating significant impacts must target as many levels within the framework as possible. For example, a person who is unconvinced about the health benefits of regular exercise (intrapersonal factor) is less likely to engage in exercise as the one who only worries about safety (community level factor) in his or her environment but believes in the value of exercise.

## DIFFUSION OF INNOVATION

The theory of Diffusion of Innovation is about spreading a new idea among a group of potential users of that idea through different communication channels that exist among the members of that group. The model owes its origins to the agricultural sector in the United States, based on the need to spread new agricultural innovations among farmers (Oldenburg et al. 1997). An innovation is a new idea, while diffusion is the means through which that idea is spread or circulated among its potential users over time.

There are two extremely critical components of this model. The first one is that adoption of the new idea, as the innovation diffuses does not happen at the same time for everybody in the group. Rather, people who adopt or take up the innovation fall within six categories known as innovators, early adopters, early majority, later majority, later adopters, and laggards (Hayden 2019). The second critical component is the idea that there are several factors that hasten the adoption of the new innovation among the users. In no particular order, some of these factors include the following:

- The extent to which the innovation fits within the social and cultural context
- How easy it is to use and how much time it will take
- Whether it is an improvement to what it replaces
- Whether it can be tried, reversed, or discontinued easily

- If the risk involved is less

Within the health sector, the diffusion and uptake of an innovation is particularly relevant when risky and unhealthy behaviors are targeted. Our world is constantly impacted by technological innovations, where healthy habits like routine visits to the doctor's office, regular physical activity, and healthy dietary habits are sacrificed for convenience and other considerations. If utilized appropriately, communication channels (formal and informal) and community role models, which are integral components of the diffusion process may help encourage positive behavioral modifications.

## THE SOCIAL SUPPORT AND SOCIAL NETWORK MODEL

One level of the Ecological Framework for health promotion and disease prevention is interpersonal level factors, which essentially refer to a person's network of social support. The social setting within which people live constitutes an enabler to people's health, which is why Heaney and Israel (1997) have concluded that "one's social relationships affect one's health" (p. 179). Therefore, it is necessary to comprehend the significance of these relationships on people's health behaviors and health outcomes. Understanding this nexus may produce support systems, especially for individuals who struggle to develop and adopt healthy behaviors and practices.

Social support is defined as "the functional content of relationships" that includes four components as follows:

- Emotional support that provides empathy and love
- Instrumental social support which deals with the provision of concrete aid and services
- Informational support that deals with giving advice and suggestions that one needs to solve problems, and
- Appraisal support which relates to constructive feedback or affirmation that may be used for self-reevaluation (House 1981).

Glanz et al distinguish social support as an approach which "focuses on one relationship at a time," and social network approach "that allows for the study of how changes in one social relationship affect other relationships" (p.182). Whether social support comes from an individual or from a network involving others in that network, the receipt of such support may benefit the recipient in improving health behaviors. For example, studies have shown that people who receive support from family members or other network members are more likely to exercise than those who do not (Kanu 2000).

This chapter, and the previous chapter, have made a cursory attempt to look at how reputable organizations such as the WHO and MSF continue to develop, refine, and share knowledge and modus operandi about health protection and disease prevention with countries across the world. These innovations or standardization of procedures have helped to refine practices that otherwise may be risky and unsafe in developing countries. Similarly, behavioral scientists through many years of research, have developed and tested behavioral change theories, models, and frameworks to guide public health practitioners and clinicians in the design and implementation of health education, health promotion, and disease prevention programs. These are efforts that must continue as new health challenges (whether due to infectious diseases or behavioral lifestyles) continue to emerge.

# *Chapter 5*

# Improving Cultural Sensitivity among Clinicians and Allied Health Professionals

Elizabeth A. Williams

Health disparities, which are defined as "a particular type of health difference closely linked with social, economic, or environmental disadvantage" are not unique to Sierra Leone or its people (Luquis and Perez 2014). With a population of over 7 million, of which 60 percent live below the poverty level, Sierra Leone is prime for experiencing the types of health differences commonly linked to disadvantage (Troslair 2020). As an example, Sierra Leone has one of the lowest life expectancies in the world, with women living an average of 54 years, while men live 52 years (World Health Organization 2020). With a fragile healthcare system made even more vulnerable by the civil war between 1991 and 2001, and the Ebola virus outbreak in 2014, the healthcare system has limited capacity to care for the health promotion and disease prevention needs of the population (Mackinnon and Maclaren 2012). With this diminished capacity of the healthcare system to provide adequate care, the health disparity burden in Sierra Leone has only increased. Similar to what is found in many developing nations, Sierra Leone and the nation's people are caught between experiencing high rates of communicable disease, compounded by growing and equally burdensome rates of non-communicable disease (Idriss et al. 2020). Illustrating this fact, the WHO estimates that the percentage of deaths from non-communicable diseases rose from 18 percent to 206 percent between 2008 and 2012 in Sierra Leone, due to increased deaths from heart disease, diabetes, and cancer (World Health Organization 2017).

While the situation described demonstrates the appalling aspect of health in Sierra Leone, and the causes for health disparities are many, there are some underlying factors that exacerbate these conditions. These include income, race and/or ethnicity, and language competence. Overwhelming evidence indicates that cultural and linguistic competencies play a significant role in reducing health disparities (Luquis and Perez 2014). As noted in this literature, lack of information about different ethnic groups, lack of culturally responsive healthcare providers, an inadequate number of healthcare professionals with diverse skills, and culturally biased healthcare services and health policies are some of the factors that have been identified as detrimental to the health status of non-White populations (Brach and Frazier 2000).

Added to these root causes of disparities are others, including variations in the preferences of patients, differences in how patients/clients recognize symptoms, and challenges in patients/clients' abilities to communicate symptoms to providers who understand their meaning. Patients from cultural backgrounds different from providers also have difficulties understanding prescribed treatments and recommended prevention strategies. Lastly, differences in patients/clients' expectations for care and challenges in adherence to preventive measures and medication regimes are additional factors that create health disparities (Betancourt et al. 2003). These factors influence patient/client and provider decision-making. They also impact interactions between patients and the health care delivery and public health system, thereby contributing to health disparities (Betancourt et al. 2003).

Cultural and linguistic competence are necessary to address health disparities at the healthcare provider and patient level for many reasons. As the National Center for Cultural Competence notes, cultural and linguistic competence are needed because beliefs about health and perceptions about health, disease, and illness vary among cultural groups. Cultural group identification also influences help-seeking behavior and attitudes toward healthcare providers. Culture also plays a role in informing people's use of traditional and complementary health practices (Goode and Dunne 2003). These aspects of culture are evident in the response in Sierra Leone to the Ebola crisis, and most recently to the COVID-19 virus pandemic. Just as cultural and linguistic incompetence can impede efforts to redress public health challenges, cultural and linguistic competence can play an important role in combating health challenges and redressing health disparities. This chapter proposes to demonstrate how providing culturally and linguistically competent care is possible in African contexts such as Sierra Leone. This chapter further outlines what cultural competency is and its benefits relative to eliminating health disparities, compares models for increasing cultural competence among health care providers and public health professionals, and describes how culturally competent health care can be provided in Africa. Case studies will be used, where appropriate, to illustrate these issues.

Cultural competence in health care and public health has been defined in multiple ways. These varied definitions include describing cultural competence as a quality health care delivery endpoint, as a behavioral and attitudinal orientation toward cross-cultural differences, and as a way of measuring how health care and public health systems use cross-cultural awareness in practice.

With an emphasis on health care delivery and outputs, cultural competence is defined as "Understanding the importance of social and cultural influences on patients' health beliefs and behaviors; considering how these factors interact at multiple levels of the health care delivery system; and finally, devising interventions that take these issues into account to assure quality health care delivery to diverse patient populations" (Betancourt et al. 2003).

Beyond fostering understanding of factors and influences that affect health outcomes with the intent of developing interventions for diverse population groups, cultural competence has also been defined as an overarching orientation or systems operational approach for responding to cross-cultural difference. As the U.S. Department of Health Resources and Services Administration defines: "Cultural competence comprises behaviors, attitudes, and policies that can come together in a continuum that will ensure that a system, agency, program, or individual can function effectively and appropriately in diverse cultural interactions and settings. It ensures an understanding, appreciation, and respect of cultural differences and similarities within, among and between groups" (p. 249S) (Selig et al. 2006). Lastly, cultural competence is defined based on how health care and public health systems use awareness of health beliefs and behaviors, disease prevalence and incidence, and treatment and outcomes for different populations (Lavizzo-Mourey and Mackenzie 1996). Each of these definitions hinge on ideas about culture and health, and interactions between them.

Expanding on the definition put forward by Cross et al. (1989), "culture" is "the integrated pattern of human behavior that includes thoughts, communications, actions, customs, beliefs, values, and institutions of racial, religious or ethnic social groups and as such are relevant to everyone's health and health care." Kleinman, Eisenberg, and Good's seminal article (1978) was among the first to articulate the importance of considering culture in health care and to demonstrate how an anthropological perspective can benefit health care delivery and outcomes. Viewed through the lens of cultural competence, health disparities such as those evidenced in Sierra Leone are more than population health challenges. They also reflect social and culture influences that have created and maintained unequal and deleterious health outcomes experienced by Sierra Leoneans. While cultural competence identifies factors that result in health disparities, greater attention to cultural competence can also suggest ways for changing these outcomes for the better.

More than a macro-level idea regarding how systems provide health care, cultural competence also involves how health professionals provide care or create policies that affect public health. The Joint Committee on Health Education and Promotion Terminology defines (2012), cultural competence as "a developmental process defined as a set of values, principles, behaviors, attitudes, and policies that enable health professionals to work effectively across racial, ethnic, and linguistically diverse groups." Emphasizing the interplay between health care systems and the people who work in them, Luquis and Perez (2003) define cultural competence as "the capacity of an individual and organization to understand, behave, and respect the values, attitudes, and beliefs of different cultural groups, and to incorporate these differences in the development and implementation and evaluation of policies and health education and promotion programs" (p. 113). Notable from both definitions, cultural competence is a developmental process that applies to both individuals and organizations.

As a developmental process, cultural competence and values and behaviors that reflect it in practice are acquired over time. In fact, cultural competence is a lifelong process. At the individual level, cultural competence requires a person to examine their own cultural values and beliefs. It also requires that a person be willing to engage in self-reflection and critique of their own biases and prejudices. Additionally, cultural competence requires the willingness of a person to expand their understanding of others and their beliefs. At the individual level, cultural competence is fundamentally a commitment to respecting the beliefs and values of other cultural groups.

Awareness of one's own biases and respect for the beliefs and values of other cultural groups requires a particular orientation in relation to others. Namely, this orientation involves cultural humility. Cultural humility includes both self-reflection and self-critique as an individual views themselves as a lifelong learner and reflective practitioner (Tervalon and Murray-Garcia 1998). As part of a commitment to lifelong learning and reflective practice, one seeking to become culturally competent, namely health care providers and public health professionals, recognize and check power imbalances and differentials that affect the quality and outcome of interactions with patients/clients and communities they serve. Health professionals exercising cultural humility, as a component of cultural competence, seek mutually respectful and dynamic partnerships with others within and across diverse cultural contexts. They also recognize that, as professionals, they do not know everything about the health concerns they seek to address or about the culture(s) of the people whose health outcomes they are working to improve. As health professionals who recognize the limits of what they do know, while appreciating the skills and knowledge they can offer, health professionals operating out of cultural humility create opportunities for learning from and working with others, including patients/clients, communities, colleagues, and others to create beneficial and sustainable responses to health needs and challenges (Tervalon and Murray-Garcia 1998).

During earlier debates about cultural competence and cultural humility, practitioners and scholars established clear distinctions between the two ideas. However, more recent scholarship has sought to reconcile these divisions and offer both as necessary for effective health practice. In synthesizing the two ideas, cultural competence is viewed as cultural knowledge transfer, whereas cultural humility is understood as a type of personal and professional selflessness necessary for cultural competence to effectively occur (Greene-Morton and Minkler 2020). As Greene-Morton further considers the two concepts, she notes cultural humility as "the ability to maintain and interpersonal stance that is other-oriented (or open to others)" (p. 144). To this she adds, cultural competence is the ability to effectively engage with people from different cultures, which is described as a "learned/taught condition" (p. 144). In summary, cultural humility is a necessary component of cultural competency because it is the attitudinal stance from which one engages with others.

Added to cultural humility, as a necessary component of cultural competence, is the further need for critical consciousness. Critical consciousness is the need to recognize how power differentials between professionals and the institutions they represent, and patients/clients and communities impact interactions and affect outputs (as policies and health interventions) and outcomes. As some scholars have critiqued, cultural competence must focus on more than interpersonal relations between people, and must deal with institutional racism and oppression at multiple levels where it exists, individually, structurally, and globally (Abrams and Moio 2009). Critical consciousness calls for interrogating how racism, classism, gender discrimination, and other forms of oppression make it possible for some groups' health and health behaviors to be hyper-scrutinized (i.e., non-White, non-Western populations) while others and their behaviors are normalized (i.e., White, Western populations) (Williams 2016). Critical consciousness, similar to that reflected in critical race theory anti-racist work, further challenges how endemic racism permeates social structures and practices, including professional training and delivery of services (Abrams and Moio 2009). Critical consciousness, paired with cultural humility and cultural competence, should challenge health professionals to recognize how their beliefs are shaped by cultural experiences and the ways in which these beliefs are helpful and detrimental to policy, practice, service delivery, and those affected by each (Williams 2016).

Having examined what cultural competence is and how it is defined, it is also important to describe how professionals learn and develop cultural competence. Also, what identifies a health professional or system as culturally competent is needed. Lastly, how cultural competence is translated into actual health practice is worthy of consideration. These ideas will be further considered.

Cultural competence as a developmental process is one that can be taught and learned by health professionals committed to individual growth and the improvement of health delivery systems and practices. Some cultural competence models explain how individuals respond to cultural differences and how responses may evolve. The Developmental Model of Intercultural Sensitivity (DMIS) and the Cultural Competence Continuum both serve as examples of this type of cultural competence model. There are also theoretical models which identify specific skills and knowledge needed to increase cultural competence. Campinha-Bacote's (2007) conceptual model of cultural competence will be described to illustrate how cultural competence is acquired to develop health care services. Finally, there are cultural competence frameworks that operationalize steps in planning health programs and interventions in culturally competent ways. The Cultural Assessment Framework (CAF), developed by Huff and Kline (1999, 2007), will be utilized to illustrate how cultural competence is applied in practice.

The Development Model of Intercultural Sensitivity (DMIS) is a cultural competence model used to explain people's responses to people who are culturally different from oneself (Paige et al. 2003). In particular, the model contains six stages, grouped according to the degree of ethnocentrism, or an individual's view of their culture as the central worldview, and ethnorelativism, or the extent one views other cultures' worldviews as being equally valid as one's own. Ethnocentric stages of the DMIS model from a greater degree of ethnocentrism to a lesser degree include denial of differences, defense of negative stereotypes of other cultures and the view of one's own culture as superior, and the minimization of differences (Diaz-Cuellar and Evans, Diversity and Health Education 2014). Ethnorelative stages of the model, in order of increasing levels of cross-cultural awareness and acceptance of diverse cultural contexts include, acceptance and respect of cultural differences, adapting a frame of reference to other cultural worldviews and lastly, integrating other world views into one's own expanding cross-cultural worldview (Diaz-Cuellar and Evans, Diversity and Health Education 2014). As one moves from one stage to another, both their attitude and behaviors should reflect greater appreciation for cultural difference and increasingly appropriate interactions and behaviors exhibited in varied cultural contexts.

Similar to the DMIS, the Cultural Competence Continuum (Goode and Jones 2004) also identifies developmental stages of cultural competence and stresses the importance of recognizing cultural competence as a dynamic process. Although as a heuristic, the Cultural Competence Continuum identifies increasing stages of cultural competence, it is not intended to present the development of cultural competence as linear. Instead, by presenting cultural competence as happening in stages, the model is intended as an assessment tool for ongoing individual self-critique and critical organizational reflection about how to achieve cultural proficiency. The Cultural Competence Continuum is a tool ideal for establishing both a baseline and benchmarks for culturally competent practice.

The first stage in the Cultural Competence Continuum is cultural destructiveness. Difference of any sort is viewed negatively and as something to eliminate. Deviations from the dominant mainstream culture are punished, suppressed, or viewed as detrimental and destructive to mainstream culture or people within these dominant cultures. In practice, cultural destructiveness is manifested as the assumed superiority of one's race, ethnicity, nationality, or culture as superior to all other cultures. Cultures other than the dominant one is viewed as inferior and those from these cultural groups are viewed as subhuman (Diaz-Cuellar and Evans, Diversity and Health Education 2014). At this stage of the continuum, the focus is on eliminating other cultures and using power and institutions to do so. Extreme examples include genocide and ethnic cleansing, forced internment, incarceration, imprisonment, deportations of asylum seekers without due process, and forced sterilization. Milder forms of cultural destructiveness include intentional exclusion of cultural groups in a health education curriculum, policies to prevent diversity, and inclusion training in institutions receiving federal funds.

Cultural incapacity is the second stage of the continuum. This stage involves seeing difference and viewing it as wrong. These views are based in the belief of one's own culture as being superior and seeks to disempower other cultures (Diaz-Cuellar and Evans, Diversity and Health Education 2014). Cultural difference, unlike in the prior stage, is not punished or suppressed. However, it is also not supported. Because the emphasis is on disempowering another's culture while elevating cultures considered to be superior, exhibited behaviors often focus on exclusion or privileging some groups while denying access or resources to others. The disproportionate allocation of resources to particular groups, expectation that "others" should change their behavior to model that of other groups, paternalism of making policies decisions for others because "others" are perceived as lacking the capacity to make decisions for themselves, and lack of equal representation of staff and administrators, who reflect the diversity of communities served are examples of cultural incapacity (Diaz-Cuellar and Evans, Diversity and Health Education 2014). The intended message conveyed whether by individuals or institutions at this stage of the continuum is that diversity and inclusion are not valued or welcome (Diaz-Cuellar and Evans, Diversity and Health Education 2014).

The third stage of the continuum is cultural blindness. Differences between cultures are seen; however, they are ignored or responded to as if they do not exist. Cultural differences are viewed as being inconsequential or as if they do not matter. No time, attention or resources are given to understanding cultural difference. Diverse populations are treated and serviced as if they are all the same. Public health program developers or practitioners do not see the need to focus on cultural issues in designing or implementing interventions or feel threatened when cultural differences are noted (Diaz-Cuellar and Evans, Diversity and Health Education 2014). The diversity of cultural groups and people are erased. Everyone is presumably viewed and treated the same way, without acknowledging biases or prejudices.

Often organizations make assumptions that everyone has access to the same resources, learns the same way, seeks services the same way, or will respond in similar ways to health information or warning. Culturally blind agencies or organizations view the dominant culture and its approaches as universally applicable to all groups and contexts, no matter how different they might be from the dominant culture (Diaz-Cuellar and Evans, Diversity and Health Education 2014). Consequently, little to no investment is made in tailoring information, services or approaches for different contexts or cultural groups. Instead, approaches and services are provided as if one size fits all.

A recognition of cultural differences, yet an inadequate response to reforming repressive structures, practices, teaching, or service approaches is indicative of the fourth stage of the model, cultural pre competence. Organizations and individuals may have an increasing awareness of how limited their skills or abilities are in interacting with or servicing diverse cultural groups. As a remedy, organizations might seek a quick fix by offering a one-time diversity workshop, hire a single member of a local diverse community as a token representative, or have a single activity in recognition of a specific cultural group (Diaz-Cuellar and Evans, Diversity and Health Education 2014). Often these efforts are recognized by others as disingenuous because there is no true commitment to diversity or inclusion, instead only superficial investment in the appearance of tolerance of cultural difference.

Cultural competence is the fifth stage of the model. At this level, individuals or organizations see cultural differences as well as recognize the effects of cultural differences. Individuals interact with people from diverse cultural groups and reflect the essential elements of cultural proficiency, including accessing culture, acknowledging differences and valuing diversity, reframing differences not in a negative light, but managing the dynamics of differences, adapting to differences and diversity, and changing practices and policies for differences (Diaz-Cuellar and Evans, Diversity and Health Education 2014). Individuals at this stage have learned to value and respect cultural differences and affirm and support differences among themselves, and seek knowledge to learn more about social injustice, privilege, and power differentials within society. Culturally competent professionals consult the diverse communities they work on behalf of and model behaviors that reflect an appreciation of cross-cultural difference. People and organizations committed to cultural competence continue self-assessment regarding culture, with careful attention to the dynamics of differences and ongoing adaptation to best serve the needs of diverse populations (Diaz-Cuellar and Evans, Diversity and Health Education 2014).

The final stage of the continuum is cultural proficiency. This stage entails identifying differences and positively responding in a supportive manner. Culture is esteemed, and learning about individual and organizational culture is valued, along with working effectively in diverse cultural environments. People who exhibit cultural proficiency recognize and respond to cultural differences and redressing oppressive structures, practice, policies, and injustice. They work for change and transformation, working in partnership with groups other than their own, differentiating the needs of people, and seek to incorporate communities and stakeholders in implementing equitable policies and services.

Cultural competence is a developmental process and is a lifelong journey to achieve equity and justice by valuing and managing cultural difference. It reflects a commitment to growth in attitudes, behaviors, policies, and practices (Diaz-Cuellar and Evans, Diversity and Health Education 2014). Culturally competent practitioners are those who become less ethnocentric and more ethnorelative in ways that benefit improved interactions with others, resulting in more effective service delivery and improved outcomes for those served by these practitioners.

While understanding cultural competence as a developmental process is necessary, it is not sufficient to guide people in becoming culturally competent professionals. Theoretical models which identify specific skills and knowledge that reflect cultural competence are needed, particularly those that are transferable to practice. These models introduce specific behaviors and orientations that people can use to increase one's self-awareness and awareness of others, along with putting cultural competence into practice. An example of this type of theoretical model is a Culturally Competent Model of Care developed by Campinha-Bacote (Campinha-Bacote, The process of cultural competence in the delivery of healthcare services: A culturally competent model of care (5th ed.), 2007). Developed to improve health care service delivery, the model identifies five essential constructs: cultural awareness, cultural knowledge, cultural skills, cultural encounters, and cultural desires. The constructs have immediate and direct applicability to professionals and their work.

Cultural awareness is a cognitive process that promotes professionals in becoming sensitive to the values, beliefs, and practices of different cultural groups (Luquis, Health Education Theoretical Models and Multicultural Populations 2014). This process includes people honestly exploring their own cultural values and background, along with a critical examination of one's biases and prejudices toward other cultural groups. For example, people may harbor biases or prejudices toward people from racial or ethnic groups, which manifest as preferential treatment toward people from favored racial/ethnic groups and disregard for people from less highly valued groups. Tools such as the Harvard University developed, Implicit Association Tests are ideal for identifying unconscious biases or prejudices people may harbor toward various markers of cultural difference, including biases toward Muslims, Native Americans and indigenous people, sexuality, gender, age, skin tone, and others. These tests also identify implicit associations people make about groups and types of behaviors (i.e., African Americans, weapons, and criminality) (Project Implicit 2020). These tests, which provide respondent's individual results, interpretation of results, and comparative analysis of a respondent's outcomes in relation to others are intended to motivate people think deeply about their feelings in response to the outcomes of these assessments. Awareness marks the first step toward changing ways of thinking or behavior that are detrimental to culturally competent practice (Campinha-Bacote 1998, 2009).

Once a person is aware of their cultural background and biases, they must be willing to undergo a process of acquiring cultural knowledge to learn more about other cultural groups worldviews. This knowledge includes understanding social and biological factors which contribute to health disparities among different racial, ethnic, and cultural groups. Reading published literature about the cultural views of various groups, taking courses to learn more about health disparities, health equity, and the history and culture of particular groups, joining professional organizations which sponsor conferences, webinars, and other educational events dealing with culture and health are readily available ways to increase cultural knowledge (Luquis 2014). Many academic degree programs in medicine and allied health disciplines further require students to take courses related to culture and health as part of their curricula (Long 2012; Like 2011; Sorensen et al. 2017).

Other state public health departments and universities, as the Maryland Department of Health and Mental Hygiene, and the University of Maryland College Park School of Public Health have developed a primer for teaching health professionals and students about cultural competency and health literacy (McCann et al. 2013). Resources such as the primer can be used in classroom settings or as a tool for individual, self-paced learning.

While the development of cultural awareness and knowledge are essential to preparing health professionals to work in diverse contexts, people also need skills to support their efforts. Cultural skills involve the ability to collect culturally relevant data and information regarding groups or individuals presented with health concerns as well as conduct assessments to determine needs and assets to develop and implement sustainable public health interventions, and evaluate the effectiveness of these interventions (Campinha-Bacote 2009). Development of cultural skills enables professionals to develop rapport with communities of interest, and access needed data to make decisions that are sensitive to the actual needs and desires of the populations for which they are intended. Skills and professional orientations inherent to disciplines like anthropology, including participant observation, interviewing, developing rapport, and the ethics of engagement, are ideal cultural skills for professionals to learn and cultivate (Bernard 2011a, 2011b; Kiefer 2006).

Professionals use of cultural skills requires engagement with people from diverse cultural backgrounds. This occurs ideally through cultural encounters (Campinha-Bacote 1998, 2009). Cultural encounters are opportunities for persons to interact directly with people from communities being served or with members of groups one is interested in learning more about. While interacting with a few members of a particular ethnic group may provide a person with increased understanding of the cultural beliefs and practices, these few encounters will not provide knowledge of all of the diverse perspectives of people who are members of a particular racial, ethnic or other cultural group. Basing one's opinions about others solely on a few encounters can easily lead to reductionist ideas about groups and stereotyping. To avoid these pitfalls, culturally competent professionals must continually seek cultural encounters with others to acquire experiential knowledge needed for appropriate health care system responses and intervention development. Professionals must also recognize there are personal limits to knowing all the varied perspectives of members of any cultural group (Greene-Morton and Minkler 2020).

For many health professionals, cultural encounters originate through opportunities to interact with colleagues, clients, patients, and people from other cultural backgrounds similar to and different from one's own (Luquis 2014). Interactions with others increases a health professionals abilities to learn from and engage with others, particularly if these encounters are engaged with cultural humility and mutual respect for others (Tervalon and Murray-Garcia 1998; Greene-Morton and Minkler 2020). The more health professionals and public health practitioners endeavor to seek out and participate in cultural encounters, the better equipped they will be in providing culturally competent responses to health concerns among diverse populations.

Having the cultural skills to have cultural encounters with diverse constituents, along with cultural knowledge and cultural awareness are important behaviors to enact to increase one's cultural competence. However, skills, knowledge, and awareness are most fruitful to practice when they are supported by cultural desire. Cultural desire is the genuine motivating force that causes a person to desire to work with people from diverse backgrounds and seek to become culturally competent (Campinha-Bacote 1998, 2009). Cultural desire is not something that can be taught in a classroom setting; it must instead be something that a professional has within themselves to seek to grow, learn, and become culturally competent (Luquis 2014). Those who approach their work from this perspective are doing a service to the populations they care for by seeking to provide culturally appropriate responses, and also to the health profession (Campinha-Bacote 1999).

To further assist professionals in measuring these constructs in practice, Campinha-Bacote, in 2003 developed the Inventory for Assessing the Process of Cultural Competence among Healthcare Professionals (IAPCC). A composite score from the subscales which measure each of the five constructs indicates a respondent's level of cultural competence that can be reasonably mapped onto Diaz-Cuellar and Evans' (2014) Cultural Competency Continnum. Higher composite scores reflect increased levels of cultural competence evidenced by the cultural proficiency (91 to 100), and culturally competent (75 to 90). Lower composite scores likewise reflect diminished levels of cultural competence, namely the cultural awareness (51 to 74) or cultural incompetence stages (25 to 50). These last two levels match closest with the stages of cultural pre competence and cultural blindness on Diaz-Cuellar & Evans' continuum (2014).

With a focus toward developing not just culturally competent practitioners but also responsive approaches to resolve health challenges, other scholars committed to cultural competence have focused their attention on developing frameworks for assessing need, developing interventions, and evaluating the outcomes of these efforts. While there are several frameworks used currently, one of the most accessible is the Cultural Assessment Framework developed by Huff and Kline (2007).

The Cultural Assessment Framework (CAF) includes domains of inquiry that are race, ethnicity, and cultural driven. Intended as a tool to drive assessment prior to developing interventions, policies or service delivery approaches, CAF should ideally be used first in driving formative evaluation. Thereafter, CAF is also an appropriate framework for informing the development and implementation of policies, strategies and approaches, along with evaluating processes and outcomes. The five categories of assessment in the framework include cultural or ethnic group-specific demographic characteristics; cultural or ethnic-group specific epidemiological and environmental influences; general and specific cultural or ethnic groups characteristics, general and specific health care beliefs and practices; and Western health care organization and service delivery variables (Huff and Kline 2007; Luquis 2014).

Cultural or ethnic groups specific demographics characteristics include gender, age, social class and status, education and literacy, religions, language, occupation and income, residence and living conditions, and acculturation or the degree to which one acquires a new cultural identity without discarding elements of one's first culture (Huff and Kline 2007, Roat et al. 1999; Diaz-Cuellar and Evans 2014). By learning as much as possible about these characteristics, health professionals can develop responses that are tailored and responsive to the needs of populations of interest. For example, in the context of Sierra Leone, it would be helpful for health professionals and public health practitioners to be cognizant of the diversity of ethnic groups represented within the country. In the survey conducted for this study, respondents identified affiliation with fourteen ethnic groups across the country. However, more than 63 percent of 583 respondents identified belonging to two ethnic groups, the Temnes (n = 206, 34.76%) and the Mendes (n = 168, 28.33%). This was similar to a 2019 National Health Survey of more than 23,000 Sierra Leonians conducted by Statistics Sierra Leone and the International Finance Corporation (IFC), in which 36 percent of women and 35 percent of men were Temne, and 31 percent of women and 30 percent of men were Mende (Statistics Sierra Leone (Stats SL) and ICF 2019). Among this study's survey respondents nearly one-half (½) had attained either secondary or university level education (n = 290, 48.91%), reflecting a relatively well educated population. Demographic characteristics like these need to be taken into consideration when developing policies, programs, and interventions targeting specific multicultural groups and subpopulations (Luquis 2014).

Population health assessment models often include epidemiological and environmental influences. Huff and Kline (2007) also recommend giving careful consideration to these factors. Only examining aggregated health data may conceal subpopulation variations that may be important for consideration and intervention. For example, a 2019 National Demographic Health survey, conducted by Statistics Sierra Leone and IFC in Sierra Leone and sponsored by the United States Agency for International Development (USAID), Global Fund, Department for International Development (DFID), United Nations Population Fund (UNFPA), World Health Organization (WHO), and the World Bank examined the knowledge of infectious disease prevention, specifically HIV prevention. 74 percent of women and 85 percent of men aged 15-49 years knew that consistent use of condoms prevents transmission of HIV, and 82 percent of women and 87 percent of men knew that limiting sexual intercourse to one faithful, uninfected partner can reduce HIV transmission (Statistics Sierra Leone (Stats SL) and ICF 2019). However, the extent of comprehensive knowledge of HIV prevention is not equally shared among younger Sierra Leoneans. Among those between 15-24 years, only 29 percent of women and 28 percent of men had comprehensive knowledge of methods to prevent HIV transmission (Statistics Sierra Leone (Stats SL) and ICF 2019). The degree to which people in this country had comprehensive knowledge of HIV prevention methods also varied based on rural versus urban residence, age, and marital status (Statistics Sierra Leone (Stats SL) and ICF 2019). Knowledge of epidemiologic differences in subgroups is key to developing appropriate interventions for populations with the greatest health need.

A hallmark of cultural competence is advocacy for health professionals and public health practitioners to become knowledgeable about specific cultural or ethnic characteristics of populations of interest (Luquis et al. 2006). These cultural or ethnic characteristics include cultural or ethnic identity, cosmology, perceptions of self and community, time orientations, social norms, values, and customs, along with communication patterns (Levy and Gaufin 2012). For example, in many African contexts, person-to-person communication often serves as a more effective way of changing health behaviors than the use of mass media. This preferred means of communication is directly related to the oral tradition, which has functioned as the bedrock for the production and acquisition of knowledge, and construction of reality in many African cultures (Airhihenbuwa 1995). Cultural and ethnic characteristics of groups are tied to the overall culture of groups, which include elements like the beliefs, practices, habits, norms, and values individuals learn from their families and communities (Spector 2004). Although people's cultural identity can change over time as people move and assimilate or acculturate to new cultural contexts, more often people's most basic cultural characteristics, as preferred communication styles remain relatively constant. Dimensions of culture, such as communication styles, form the basis of people's cultural identity, which consequently influence people's health choices and behaviors (Huff and Kline 2007). Awareness of these cultural and ethnic characteristics supports the development and implementation of policies and approaches that align with the cultural characteristics of the populations for which they are developed. Lack of awareness of cultural and ethnic characteristics can result in policies and practices that are contrary to predominant characteristics and creates barriers to health promotion, disease prevention, and health service delivery that exacerbate rather than remedy health challenges.

As part of the Cultural Assessment Framework, health professionals and public health practitioners should be mindful of specific racial and ethnic health care beliefs and practices which can affect a group's interaction with the Western biomedical model or health promotion efforts (Huff and Kline 2007). Knowledge of these beliefs and practices would include assessment of group's health and illness explanatory models, responses to illness, perceptions and use of Western health care and health promotion services, and health-seeking behaviors. The Western biomedical model explains illness and sickness in terms of disease and pathological agents; whereas, many ethnic or other cultural groups explain illness, disease, or treatment from a cultural or social perspective different from that of Western biomedicine's point of view. (Jones 1994; Edberg 2013; Kiefer 2006) Ethnic or cultural groups that adhere to personalistic ethnomedical systems may view ill health as the cause of sorcery, spells or the intervention of supernatural agents (Edberg 2013). As a consequence, treatment will entail blocking or countering spiritual or supernatural forces.

Suggestive of ethnic health care beliefs and practices in Sierra Leone that are similar to and differ from the Western biomedical model, the survey conducted for this book asked respondents to indicate which treatment modalities they believed in for healing. Respondents were permitted to indicate all that applied; therefore, total responses summed to be more than 100 percent. Of the options provided, 90 percent of respondents (n=534) indicated clinical medicine, 272 respondents (45.87%) indicated that traditional healers/medicine were also believed effective for healing, and 243 responses (40.98%) affirmed spiritual healing as effective. Moray-man and the use of charms, along with fortune-tellers/sorcerers were indicated by 50 (8.43%) and 37 (6.24%) respondents, respectively. These responses indicate that members of ethnic and cultural groups in Sierra Leone may be as likely to follow a non-Western treatment modality to deal with disease or illness, as they would be to visit a Western biomedical health provider or use Western biomedical treatments. Sierra Leoneans' medically syncretic approach to healthcare seeking and health care beliefs reflect the importance of health professionals and public health practitioners being aware of ethnic and cultural groups' understanding of health and illness, health beliefs and practices, and their willingness to incorporate cultural groups' views into health interventions (Luquis 2014).

The Cultural Assessment Framework finally proposes that the Western health care organization and public health delivery systems that provide services to multicultural groups must also be assessed (Huff and Kline 2007). How the health care organization or system perceives and works with the groups it serves is a key component of assessment (Huff and Kline 2007). This assessment would include an assessment of the cultural competence of the health professionals and public health practitioners providing services, an assessment of the organization's mission and policies that promote cultural competence, and an assessment of the evaluative processes in place to measure an organization's efforts in these areas (Luquis 2014).

The Sierra Leone government's Ministry of Health and Sanitation published the Health Sector Recovery Plan, 2015–2020, which included a situational analysis of the country's response to the Ebola outbreak in 2014 (Ministry of Health and Sanitation 2015). One of the noted areas of concern in response to the infectious disease outbreak was the lack of skilled health professionals. Although 13,000 community health workers, paraprofessionals from local communities, were dispersed to provide nutritional, family planning, and other non-clinical services—these essential health workers functioned as volunteers and were never formally instituted as part of the health sector. Additionally, in response to the Ebola outbreak, these community health workers were not trained to provide health education, that could have been vital to informing people throughout the country of Ebola prevention strategies to mitigate disease spread (Ministry of Health and Sanitation 2015).

As part of the service delivery system assessment, the Ministry of Health and Sanitation's Plan also outlines key priority areas as part of the Health Sector Recovery Framework. One of the identified areas is Community Ownership. Key strategies include to:

- Ensure community groups of key stakeholders (dialogue structures including women and youth) and networks are established and systematically engaged in BPEHS implementation;
- Ensure key community groups and networks are engaged in community surveillance, case investigation and other key operational events; and
- Ensure key policies, strategies, and guidelines on community engagement are developed to support the implementation of the BPEHS (Ministry of Health and Sanitation 2015).

The Sierra Leone Ministry of Health's recognition of the need to include communities in the process of assessing and delivering health services reflects the Cultural Assessment Framework's call for Western health care organization and service delivery systems to evaluate their efforts to enhance cultural competence. As an example, the Health Sector Recovery Plan explicitly includes the need for creating strong linkages between health systems and communities to promote behavior change around isolation, and safe burials of persons infected with Ebola. It also cites working with traditional leaders to enforce local by-laws and decrees, along with religious groups, women's groups, and youth groups as effective strategies in demonstrating political commitment to address the epidemic and enhance the effectiveness of prevention messaging, and mobilization of populations regarding the use of health care services. Lastly, using neighborhood watch programs and community surveillance were also cited as a major contribution toward active surveillance and early detection and referral of infected persons for treatment and care (Ministry of Health and Sanitation 2015).

As reflected by the Sierra Leone Ministry of Health's Plan, health care systems and public health are increasingly becoming aware of the importance of culture in redressing population health challenges, especially public health emergencies like the Ebola outbreak in Sierra Leone, and surrounding West African nations in 2014-2016. While this chapter is focused on defining cultural competence, describing cultural competence theoretical models for individual and organizational assessment, and outlining the Cultural Assessment Framework as a tool for assessing cultural characteristics, influences, beliefs and practices, and organizational and service delivery variables, that can support culturally competent health care and public health delivery—it is only fitting to highlight an example of a health system and public health intervention which reflects these ideas in practice. The Social Mobilization Action Consortium (SMAC), a large-scale community engagement intervention implemented in Sierra Leone to support Ebola outbreak containment, serves as an example of this type of culturally competent practice.

The SMAC was established in September 2014 as an effort by five partner organizations, including GOAL, an international humanitarian response agency; Restless Development Sierra Leone, an international development agency; FOCUS 1000, a Sierra Leonean non-governmental organization; BBC Media Action, an international development charity; and the U.S. Centers for Disease Control and Prevention. The intervention's intents were to train and support communities in Sierra Leone to implement community action plans to mitigate the spread of Ebola and support improved health care system utilization among community members in response to the disease.

The SMAC intervention grew out of a national assessment conducted in August 2014 to determine the public's knowledge, attitudes, and practices within Sierra Leone (Jalloh et al. 2017). Similar to the CAF's emphasis on assessing cultural and ethnic-group specific epidemiological and environmental influences (Huff and Kline 2007), the national assessment revealed a high level of awareness and knowledge about Ebola in Sierra Leone, along with misconceptions, stigma, and other identified barriers to disease mitigation (Jalloh et al. 2017). Anthropological research conducted early during the outbreak identified general health care beliefs and practices shared among Sierra Leoneans to address the disease and reflected this domain of the Cultural Assessment Framework (Huff and Kline 2007).

This anthropological research indicates that Sierra Leoneans were willing to change their behaviors and accept emergency response measures to prevent the spread of Ebola if these measures were implemented in culturally and socially acceptable ways and were sustainable (Richards et al., 2015, Fairhead, 2014, Abramowitz et al., 2017). Sierra Leoneans' willingness to adopt preventive measures regarding safe burials reflected not a rejection of Western biomedical ideas about disease but something different. Namely, Sierran Leoneans' willingness to change their behavior, yet failure to do so initially during the outbreak reflected a critique of Western health care and public health's early disease emergency messaging and response. These early messages emphasized Ebola as a "killer disease," fell short of offering actionable strategies on prevention, treatment, and disease survival (Moon et al., 2015). The heavy-handed emphasis on fear and lack of cultural sensitivity in emergency response to community values and traditions among Sierra Leoneans about caring for ill persons and burial preparation contributed to people's reluctance to use health care services and hiding from authorities (Jalloh et al., 2017).

As the CAF's creators recognize, health care and public health systems lack of cultural competence affect service utilization within the communities these systems seek to serve. Seeking to implement an intervention that would address these issues, SMAC utilized the Community-led Ebola Action (CLEA) approach as its community engagement strategy (Bedson et al. 2020). This approach used culturally and context sensitive strategies developed by the partnering groups, reflecting a culturally competent approach to intervention development and implementation. The CLEA approach emphasizes varied ways of understanding illness, allowance for multiple simultaneous framings of disease, rather than an exclusive privileging of Western biomedical ideas, recognition of community members as experts, and rejection of ethnocentric assumptions about cultural beliefs as problems and barriers to be overcome by health care and public health systems, and communities as needing to be convinced to adopt Western biomedical approaches. The CLEA approach instead championed community responses as those which can lessen poor health outcomes and enhance health, as well as affirm adapting services to meet the needs of communities (Social Mobilisation Action Consortium 2014).

SMAC trained 2,500 mobilizers to work in communities to assist with designing and implementing community action planning. Over 6,000 religious leaders from more than 2000 mosques and churches were engaged to promote essential prevention and response messages and to role model behaviors promoted through community plans, including those regarding safe burials. More than 40 local radio stations in 14 districts across Sierra Leone were deployed to broadcast messages, and ensure synchronization and quality of radio programming related to the intervention. Mobilizers were recruited from local communities and included those with backgrounds as community health workers, development organization youth volunteers, and trusted community members. Ebola survivors were also recruited as mobilizers to bring the first-hand experiences of those impacted into the response efforts. Engaging community members as paid public health paraprofessionals, trusted leaders, and community assets into the design of the intervention—all reflect important dimensions of cultural competence, including cultural awareness and cultural knowledge (Campinha-Bacote 2007).

Mobilizers were trained in community mobilization for health and provided refresher trainings, action learning, and other capacity-building activities as part of their preparation to implement the CLEA approach. Specifically mobilizers were trained to emphasize community identification of priority actions for community action plans based on the responsiveness of the community to develop an action plan. This investment in training mobilizers to engage with community members as part of the intervention reflects an important aspect of cultural competence, specifically the development of cultural skills (Campinha-Bacote 2007). These cultural skills, along with mobilizers' participation in CLEA activities, provided opportunities for cultural encounters with communities impacted by Ebola (Campinha-Bacote 2007).

SMAC's use of the CLEA approach emphasized a two-way approach to communication and messaging within Sierra Leone about Ebola, rather than a one-way approach to the disease. This one-way health communication messaging strategy used during the early phases of the outbreak focused on the disease itself, often to the exclusion of people for which the messages were intended. Many people in countries affected by Ebola found this one-way messaging approach off-putting (Dubois et al. 2015). SMAC approached communication and messaging about the disease in two ways, namely by using an interactive and iterative community approach focused on "triggering events," as the catalyst for developing community action plans and by operationalizing a national, systematic feedback mechanism for connecting communities through recurring visits, access to a closed user mobile phone network, and providing 24-hour support to mobilizers (Bedson et al. 2020). The CLEA approach went beyond encouraging safe Ebola behaviors to creating reliable and sustainable communications infrastructure to promote information sharing between large numbers of communities, mobilizers, SMAC staff, and health system and public health response authorities (Bedson et al. 2020).

These CLEA triggering events were participatory activities intended to create a sense of urgency and facilitate communities in undertaking their own appraisal of the Ebola outbreak, its current impact on the community and the likely impact of taking no action (Bedson et al. 2020). Triggering events consisted of activities like body mapping; danger discussions; burial role-plays; personal protective equipment demonstrations; Ebola survivor stories; and Ebola spread exercises (Social Mobilisation Action Consortium 2020). Burial role-play triggering events were used to explore what a typical burial in a community might entail, along with the experience of dealing with burial response teams. During these events facilitated group discussions led by mobilizers, resulted in the development of community action plans and identification of "Community Champions," influential community members who served as focal points for program activities for the action plan (Bedson et al. 2020). Action plans often resulted in community bylaws; for example, governing entrance and exit from a community during an Ebola outbreak, which were then implemented within communities and supported by champions.

Quantitative and qualitative data on the implementation, achievement and outcomes of community action plans were gathered by mobilizers. These data were primarily collected through standardized paper forms developed for this purpose. Digital data reporting was introduced later into the intervention to document the activities of religious groups and radio stations in a representative sample of districts. Data points included actions taken, number of community visits conducted by mobilizers, mobilizers meetings and alerts broadcast, and specific activities of religious leaders and radio stations. Behavioral outcomes were measured, including timely referrals of sick household members for medical care, and timely requests of safe burials for deceased family members (Bedson et al. 2020).

CLEA's reach in communities throughout Sierra Leone was significant. Mobilizers worked with more than 12,000 communities across the country, engaging more than 2 million community members, of which 50.2 percent were women, 49.8 percent were men, and 46 percent were young people under the age of 18 years old (Bedson et al. 2020). Based on Bedson et al.'s analysis (2020) of impact, an increase over time was reflected in the fraction of community members reporting Ebola cases for medical referral within 24 hours of onset of symptoms. Monitoring data indicated that 100 percent of communities developed action plans, with an average of three action points. When digital monitoring was fully operational between April and September 2015, more than 85 percent of action plans were in progress, while 7 percent were indicated as achieved, and 7 percent were categorized as not achieved. Priorities for community action plans also shifted over time and in response to changing needs. Early during the outbreak, action plans, as reflected in bylaws, focused on community isolation and restricting movement into and out of communities as ways to reduce Ebola transmission; however, these restrictions started to decline between November 2014 and December 2015, and an uptick in bylaws regarding the handling of dead bodies and handwashing occurred during this same period (Bedson et al. 2020).

Important lessons learned from the SMAC model and its use are that behavioral interventions are more likely effective when a combination of communication strategies are used, including interpersonal communication and mass media, along with working with government strategies that are culturally tailored to meet the needs of the populations served. The CLEA approach used in this case study also demonstrates that communities and their members can be and are the most effective agents of change in response to health concerns affecting their communities. While people are influenced by their primary culture, this does not mean that people are not amiable to cultural or behavioral change. As evidenced in this example, communities are willing to change even deeply held, cultural practices when they are equipped to arrive at locally appropriate and acceptable changes in response to health threats that reflect their cultural values (Abramowitz et al. 2015). Additionally, when health care and public health systems and professionals commit to being culturally competent, practice cultural humility, and exhibit critical consciousness in how they engage with diverse populations in the design, implementation and evaluation of health strategies results often reveal better outcomes than what would be achieved without the commitment to cultural competence.

Cultural competence is not a single, quick-fix solution to redress health challenges or eliminate health disparities, experienced by medically underserved and vulnerable populations. Cultural competence, whether as an idea, a theoretical model, or an assessment framework is not designed to do this. Nevertheless, cultural competence is essential to improving population health outcomes and achieving equity in health care delivery and public health policies, interventions, and practice. Cultural competence is essential because it recognizes that culture and cultural differences matter, not as impediments to achieving optimal health, but instead as vehicles to drive greater awareness, deeper discovery, innovation, and problem solving in health. Culture matters because it influences how people understand health and illness and response. Culture matters because it shapes how health professionals interact with patients and clients and how they operate systems that impact people's health. Culture matters, and because culture matters, cultural competence is not an addendum to health professional practice. It is the cornerstone of providing care and interventions that places people and their health first.

## *Chapter 6*

# Recommendations for Best Practices

Elizabeth A. Williams

Culture involves a complex mix of what we believe, what we create, and how we interact with others. As such, culture is not one thing, but many things. At the core of people's culture are their beliefs and values. These are the cornerstones of culture. Culture is shaped by families of origin and extended family ties, natural environments, social, political, and economic contexts, experiences, history, and social interactions passed down over time and between generations. Culture forms the core structure and shape of people's lives, including their beliefs about health. Although culture is stable, this does not mean that it is immutable to change. With new information and experiences, along with changing contexts, components of culture can change among groups of people.

Both the resiliency and mutability of culture are evidenced clearly in relation to health. Individuals' beliefs and groups' collective ideas about health reflect notions about human universals, such as life and death. Cultural beliefs about health also reflect philosophical, theological, and cosmological ideas about the origin of life, order of the world, and the nature of human interactions. As a result, a group's beliefs about health, and peoples' responses to health issues reveal much about key aspects of a group's culture. Recognizing the source of these beliefs and behaviors and seeking to understand how they are shaped by culture form the basis of cultural competence.

In the context of Sierra Leone and the adjacent countries that make up the Mano River Basin region (i.e., Guinea, Liberia), the influence of culture on health and health behaviors is apparent (see figure 6.1).

With over sixteen (16) distinct ethnic groups in Sierra Leone alone, there are distinct health beliefs between groups. For example, the Fula ethnic group distinguishes between illnesses based on where they occur in the body. Illnesses that occur below the waist may be viewed as those resulting from

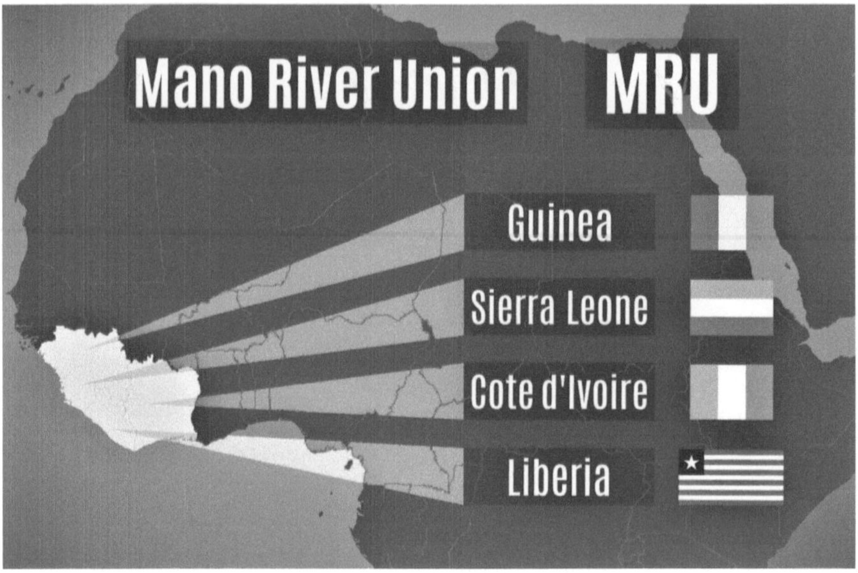


**Figure 6.1 Mano River Basin Map.** Adobe Stock. *Source:* Adobe Stock, Extended License, Adobe.com, purchased 2021.

lack of obedience to Fulani cultural traditions, rather than as consequence to exposure to a pathogen or some other etiologic cause. As a result, seeking treatment for illnesses below the waist from biomedical practitioners may be less often sought (Gordon 2000).

Just as there are distinct cultural beliefs about health among ethnic groups in Sierra Leone and surrounding countries, there are also commonly shared ideas between ethnic groups. Members of ethnic groups such as the Mende, Mandingo, and Krio utilize Western medicine in the treatment of ailments; however, they do so along with utilizing traditional healers and religious leaders for treatment. This syncretic approach to treatment seeking is not uncommon throughout the region and across the world, particularly in contexts where people have exposure and access to both Western biomedical and non-Western treatments and practitioners. The degree to which familiarity and trust of different types of treatments, practices, and practitioners exists determines whether people utilize these in response to illness. To be effective in providing care, health, and public health systems, as well as those who work in them must be aware of these dynamics and work to address them in policies and practices related to health.

The Mano River Basin region, which contains the countries of Sierra Leone, Liberia, and Guinea have recently experienced their share of social and public health challenges. Emerging in the 1980s with the spread of the Human Immunodeficiency Virus (HIV) to the present, 2020, with the

COVID-19 pandemic, this region has dealt with communicable disease outbreaks that have been unprecedented in scope and impact. The Ebola outbreak of 2014–2016 was no exception.

Several factors exacerbated the spread and devastating impact of the disease within the region. Specifically, among them were the fluidity of borders between the countries and ethnic variability within these countries. The movement of people across geographic borders between ethnic groups, along with robust trade relationships within these countries, created the ideal circumstances for the spread of the Ebola virus. Coupled with health systems that had been severely fractured by civil wars in Liberia and Sierra Leone, and political unrest in Guinea throughout the 1980s and 1990s—the political and social climate alone created the ideal social vector for disease spread (Wilkerson and Fairhead 2017).

With the rapid spread of the Ebola virus within the region, the responses of the health care and public health systems were justifiably focused on treatment of the sick, control of disease spread, and mitigating the impact of the virus. Several factors affected these systems' abilities to effectively achieve these ends, which included limited knowledge at the time about the etiology of the disease, and what behaviors increased the risk of exposure and disease transmission. Another major factor was lack of understanding about cultural value systems, practices, and how these would shape people's responses to the Ebola outbreak (Abramowitz et al. 2017; Jalloh et al. 2017).

There is an appreciation among medical anthropologists and those who work in global health contexts for the ways that culture and social context affect health practices and population health outcomes. This appreciation for cultural values, social context, and the extent of their influence is not always reflected in health care or public health practices. Such was the case with Ebola in the context of Sierra Leone and throughout the Mano River Basin region between 2014 –2016.

Part of the overarching worldview of many Africans, particularly West Africans, is the prominence of family and extended family ties. Family functions are the core of human relationships for many Sub-Saharan Africans, including those in Sierra Leone and adjacent counties. Family is the nucleus for exchange, including informational, social, and material support through the sharing of goods and services. Families rally together in times of need, and celebrate together in times of joy and triumph (Wilkerson and Fairhead 2017).

As the nexus of human relationships for many Africans, in times of crisis, extended family becomes even more pivotal. Families among many ethnic groups in Sierra Leone and throughout the Mano River Basin region are expected to care for the sick among them and assembly when people are ill. When people die, it is additionally expected that people will touch the deceased person's body as a sign of care and respect. Without knowing that the Ebola virus would spread through human contact with infected persons, including after their demise, many Sierra Leonians, and others in the region, were unknowingly at heightened risks through their adherence to cultural practices involving the sick and dying.

In addition to caring for the sick and dying, many Sierra Leoneans were put at greater risk of contracting the Ebola virus by handling and preparing the bodies of dying and deceased loved ones. With the virus easily transmissible through blood and bodily fluids, even several days after death, many contracted the disease in their efforts to prepare corpses for honorable burials. Others were also exposed by hiding or moving loved ones between relatives to care for them and/or to reduce the risk of relatives and family members being shunned because of a person's Ebola positive status (Jalloh et al. 2017; Southall et al. 2017).

What also caused some Sierra Leoneans to be at risk during the Ebola outbreak was the reliance on alternative and traditional healers. Due to the lack of trust in biomedical practitioners, cost, or concerns about care unresponsive to the needs of people, some Sierra Leoneans were reluctant to use the health care or public health sectors in response to Ebola. Instead, they sought Ebola cures from traditional healers, but these remedies were often ineffective. In part due to a lack of coordination between health and public health systems and traditional healers, people in Sierra Leone and in the Mano River Basin region seeking care often did not receive the appropriate care needed to treat the virus or information to prevent its spread (Southall et al. 2017). These circumstances resulted in missed opportunities to prevent the virus' spread and the deaths of thousands in Sierra Leone and the region.

Excluding traditional healers, alternative medical approaches, and cultural practices was not the answer to control the spread of the Ebola virus between 2014–2016 in the Mano River Basin region. It only increased people's risk of virus exposure and death. Rather than excluding traditional medicine, practitioners, and cultural practices, the story of the 2014–2016 Mano River Basin Ebola epidemic exposed the need to integrate cultural adaptations into disease prevention and treatment. The WHO and others developed approaches recognizing the importance of these factors to guide practice (World Health Organization 2014).

While what has happened cannot be undone, it can be learned from. Lessons learned can provide the blueprint to develop better and more effective responses for the next public health crisis, which is the intent of this book. It is intended to serve as a guide for practitioners and policy makers alike to create systems and responses that can more effectively treat people, prevent them from becoming sick, and that are sustainable and replicable, and culturally relevant.

In response to public health crises, such as the 2014–2016 Mano River Basin Ebola outbreak, there is increasing recognition of the important role of cultural competence. While there are multiple definitions of cultural competence, at a minimum, cultural competence involves, "Understanding the importance of social and cultural influences on patients' health, beliefs, and behaviors; considering how these factors interact at multiple levels of the health care delivery system; and finally, devising interventions that take these issues into account to assure quality health care delivery to diverse patient populations" (Betancourt et al. 2003).

Earlier chapters in this book have described what cultural competence is and how it connects to culture and health. The book also provides theoretical and conceptual models of how cultural competence can be developed by individual practitioners, and within systems and organizations. It has further offered examples of how cultural competence has been used in practice to develop health system and public health strategies in response to Ebola. Now, what remains is to offer some recommendations for how culturally competent health and public health systems and their practitioners can further translate these insights into policy and practice guidance for populations in the Mano River Basin region and beyond.

The national response to the Ebola outbreak in Sierra Leone recognized early on the need to incorporate communities in the response and create linkages between the nation's health care and public health systems, and affected populations. Rather than thwarting local politics, the Sierra Leone Ministry of Health and Sanitation's Health Sector Recovery Plan, 2015–2020, incorporated local leaders into the country's national response to the Ebola outbreak in 2014 (Ministry of Health and Sanitation 2015). Principally, the response effort built on chiefdom authority as a way to embed public health policies into locally trusted institutions (Wilkerson and Fairhead 2017).

The chiefdom structure of indigenous rulers who retain sovereignty in local affairs, and work in tandem with national political authorities is part of a bifurcated system of governance set up by the British under colonialism (Jackson 2007). Chiefdom authority for most Sierra Leonians is viewed as reflective of established cultural patterns of legitimate ritual and political authority because chiefs are elected to power through claims to ancestry. Chiefs are perceived as leaders whose interests are in the service of the people they govern. Chiefdoms operate in relation to other society leaders, including religious leaders and those within secret societies, and at times, chiefdom authority may be enhanced by overlap between society leaders and national political authority. National political authorities rely on chiefs to secure votes for general elections and chiefs depend on national politicians for resources to distribute within local communities (Jackson 2007). Rather than subverting this political structure, Sierra Leone's Ebola response capitalized on it in some important ways.

As part of the national response plan, a National Ebola Response Center (NERC) was established. With the Sierra Leonean Army responsible for logistics and enforcing quarantines, curfews and travel restrictions, this response was further supported by the British Army, which provided technical and operational support. Established based on thematic pillars, that included case management, burials, social mobilization, surveillance and others, deployment of these functions was replicated in each district of Sierra Leone through District Ebola Response Centers (DERCs) (Wilkerson and Fairhead 2017). The DERCs were administrated by Sierra Leonean and British Army personnel, civil servants from the UK Department of International Development, and Paramount Chiefs. Although the response was militarized, inclusion of chiefdoms made the response apparatus and approach more palatable to the nation's citizenry.

Chiefdom taskforces were set up in local districts, appointed by chiefs, to carry out necessary disease outbreak control activities including house to house visits, disease prevention education, and surveillance. These taskforce teams worked in conjunction with the DERC teams to implement chiefdom bylaws, which had been imposed to prevent disease transmission through restrictions on traditional funeral rites and caring for infected persons at home. These chiefdom bylaws became an essential part of the national response plan, and the President of Sierra Leone required all chiefs to impose these bylaws or risk being fined or removed if they did not enforce bylaws (Wilkerson and Fairhead 2017).

Further illustrating the power of chiefs in the Sierra Leone Ebola response effort, Ebola Community Care Centers (CCCs) were built primarily in chiefdoms. Of the 54 centers built, most were located on community donated land and were built with labor provided by local community members (Oosterhoff et al. 2015). The Ebola response intervention approach and the institutions primarily responsible for implementing it, namely chiefs and the military, were not completely unproblematic in Sierra Leone. One of the principal complaints was that jobs related to the response effort often went to those with ties to the chief, instead of being more equitably distributed among community members. (Wilkerson and Fairhead 2017). Nevertheless, the approach, which included chiefs, traditional healers, women's and youth leaders, elders, and international partners, was considered acceptable and occurred without significant contestation.

The Sierra Leonean Ebola response was qualitatively different from the approach in Guinea. Among people in the Mano River region, response to illness is informed by presumed etiology. Sudden sickness and death, which are sequela common with Ebola, are often associated with unnatural occurrences, which are understood to be the consequence of a social fault or curse (Wilkerson and Fairhead 2017). Constructed as a disease of immorality, the initial public health Ebola response in Guinea focused on educating populations about Ebola risks in the Forest Region (the area of highest initial incidence) in ways that fed into stereotypes about people, who principally followed traditional practices and participated in secret initiation societies, rather than professed Christianity or Islam. For many in Guinea, including those who are Islamic, those affiliated with the White Christian world, and African nationalists, the social and religious practices of the Forestiers were disdained (Wilkerson and Fairhead 2017).

The hypervigilance of sensitizing forest region communities to the exclusion of other populations also at high-risk, including Imams and Muslim healers involved in healing and funerals, contributed to the spread of the disease within the country. Stigmatization of those in the Forest Region as immoral created a false dichotomy between them and other populations, including Muslims and Muslim clerics who perceived themselves as morally well. This false dichotomy made it difficult for some Muslims, particularly Imams and Muslim healers, to acknowledge their susceptibility to contracting or spreading Ebola (Wilkerson and Fairhead 2017). As a result, Imams continued to wash bodies and perform other funeral rites after initial disease control efforts were underway. One even traveled to neighboring Mali by avoiding checkpoints, presumably introducing the disease within this country (Penney and Farge 2014). This segmented approach to disease control also led to resistance and resentment of some Forest Region inhabitants with being cast as immoral due to Ebola.

The way the Ebola response in Guinea was implemented was problematic in several ways. In the Guinean context, civil servants from areas historically antagonist to where the Ebola outbreak first occurred were responsible for implementing disease control efforts. With no formal ties to the communities most affected by Ebola, residents viewed the disease control efforts of externally appointed civil servants with skepticism and suspicion. The messaging of disease control education efforts principally cast the disease as an ethnic disease among residents of the Forest Region or the Kissi, which further exacerbated resentment and led to concerns about disease control measures being used to suppress Forest Region communities (Wilkerson and Fairhead 2017).

With a response led by civil servants and leaders viewed as openly critical of the Forest Region, people from locally affected areas further charged the Guinean government and its leaders with discrimination in not hiring local people for administrative appointments related to the control efforts (Wilkerson and Fairhead 2017). When a delegation of political elites, including the Governor of the Forest Region, and those who were intolerant of initiation societies arrived in a Forest Region community at a time that coincided with a presentation ceremony for girl initiates into an initiation society, tensions steeped. Having sprayed bleach over the area as part of the delegation's activities, local residents assumed that the community was being infected and residents responded by killing members of the delegation, until the Guinean military intervened (Brittian 2015). This example and others of active resistance in Guinea demonstrate how fear, resistance, and noncompliance to disease control efforts are exacerbated when there is distrust of political leaders and those leading control efforts (Fairhead 2015).

The contrasting examples of Ebola control efforts in Sierra Leone and Guinea described here point out the critical need for cultural competence in developing response policy and executing response efforts. These examples demonstrate the need for critical consciousness of the historical context in which public health crises occur. Within the Sierra Leonean context, chiefs have been historically vested with power and authority by the people, and therefore, were not viewed with suspicion when they became involved in response activities. Additionally, chiefs worked in concert with government officials as a part of a coordinated set of policies to control disease spread. Comparatively, Guineans were unable to trust externally imposed civil servants designated as responsible for implementing Ebola control measures. In the latter instance, lack of critical consciousness about the political configuration of Ebola response served as a major impediment to response activities. Also, the perceived and apparent hostility and cultural disdain of civil servants toward populations in the Forest Region further served to impede efforts (Wilkerson and Fairhead 2017).

In addition to the need for critical consciousness and an appreciation for the historical context of public health crisis response activities, there are other culturally competent recommendations for public health policymakers and health service practitioners to consider in response to Ebola and similar public health crises in Sierra Leone and the Mano River Basin region. These recommendations include:

- Reviewing culturally competent information and guidance developed by anthropologists about Ebola, and the cultural contexts of populations affected by the illness such as those available on the Ebola Response Anthropology Platform (Ebola Response Anthropology Platform, 2020);
- Engaging highly qualified African experts within the region and across the world for their scientific and professional expertise in epidemiological surveillance and developing robust public health and health system response approaches;
- Conducting cultural framework assessments by aptly trained persons to identify contextual issues and nuances needed for implementing effective

control and response activities prior to developing policies and enacting efforts (Huff and Kline 2007);

- Gaining awareness of the cultural perceptions of illness and disease among populations served by response activities;
- Recognition and acknowledgment of policy makers and response actors' biases, and how these may influence the development and implementation of response policies;
- Attention given to systemic forms of oppression (e.g., racism, xenophobia, elitism), and how these are manifested in government, public health, and health service systems in ways that perpetuate disadvantage among some populations (e.g., discriminatory hiring policies) and advantage others;
- Careful consideration given to how illness risk and populations affected by illness are constructed in policies to avoid stigmatizing socially, ethnically or politically vulnerable populations (Williams, 2016);
- Equitization of risk in response communication, education, and sensitization activities to include all populations susceptible to illness and disease, and not just hypervigilance of some populations to the exclusion of others (Williams 2016; Abrams and Moio 2009);
- Development of prevention and control strategies that are appropriate to the context of greatest need and for populations at greatest risk;
- Tailoring of health communication messages to reflect not only individual risk, but also underscore community and population risk, and offer prevention and control strategies that are logical and are applicable to the most vulnerable populations;
- Careful attention given to spokespersons chosen to render response communication to ensure that the messenger's perceived and/or real biases do not impede the impact of control and prevention messages;
- Inclusion of persons from affected areas and those perceived as credible in all aspects of response planning, coordination, implementation, and evaluation to increase buy-in and compliance with response activities;
- Educating, empowering, and appropriately compensating local community members and paraprofessionals as health educators to sensitize community members about low-cost and sustainable control measures, such as those documented by the London School of Hygiene & Tropical Medicine (London School of Hygiene and Tropical Medicine 2020);
- Incorporation of traditional healers, religious leaders, community leaders, and members of vulnerable and socially marginalized groups (e.g., women, youth) in response planning, education, implementation, and evaluation activities; and
- Equitable distribution of fiscal resources by governments and non-governmental organizations to those participating in local and regional response activities.

While this list of recommendations is not exhaustive, these recommendations, nevertheless, speak to the comprehensive need for cultural competence in all aspects of public health crisis response. The Ebola outbreak of 2014–2016 in the countries of the Mano River Basin region, including Sierra Leone, Guinea, and Liberia, continues to provide invaluable lessons for disease outbreak response in this area, throughout Sub-Saharan Africa, and across the world. As the recent COVID-19 global pandemic has underscored the need for multisectoral approaches to response, which include culturally competent perspectives, is recognized, public health scholars are calling for the development of COVID-19 communication to Black and Brown communities across the world that incorporate culturally competent theoretical models in the design of messages, as the PEN-3 model. These scholars further call for framing risk and risk reduction strategies in culturally appropriate ways, including those that emphasize community risk, which is more relevant for populations that value communal and extended family ties, rather than exclusively focusing on individual risk, which reflects a Western orientation to illness and disease (Airhihenbuwa et al. 2020).

The importance of culturally competent practitioners as part of public health crisis response is also being recognized across the continent of Africa. Presidents of many African nations have established national COVID-19 taskforces, bringing together experts from multiple sectors to craft response policy. For example, in Uganda, a Presidential Scientific and Strategic Advisory Committee includes not only public health experts, along with virologists and epidemiologists, but also anthropologists and economists to design effective policies and interventions to address the crisis (Africa Center for Strategic Studies 2020).

Additionally, concerted efforts have been undertaken by the governments of Sierra Leone, Guinea, and Liberia in response to COVID-19 based on lessons learned from the 2014–2016 Ebola crisis and the resilience developed from the experience. Having recognized early that implementing long-term stay-in-place measures were not sustainable in the economic and social context of the Mano River Basin region where people rely on trade and exchange, these governments have implemented measures to reduce community and individual risk. These control measures focus on encouraging use of locally produced masks to prevent disease transmission, instituting government placed handwashing stations across the country, encouraging the implementation of handwashing and hand sanitizer stations outside of businesses and other high traffic areas, providing water and electric subsidies for citizens, and securing borders, as occurred in Guinea's capitol city of Conakry from the rest of the country to reduce disease spread (Haken and Fiertz 2020). These COVID-19 response measures within this region build on the response networks established during the Ebola outbreak (Haken and Fiertz 2020).

The nature of public health crises across the world requires increasingly thoughtful, scientifically sound, and relevant approaches to prevent disease spread and preserve the public's health. Because public health crises affect people and the places where they work, pray, play, grow, and live, particular attention must be given to interventions that are designed by the people and fit the contexts where they live. Responding to public health crises calls for understanding how people, their behaviors, and the systems they create operate in ways that affect health outcomes. This understanding emanates through paying attention to culture and utilizing the perspectives and tools of cultural competence to influence people, culture, and contexts in ways that reduce illness risk and promote health.

# Bibliography

Abramowitz, S., McKune, S. L., Fallah, M., Monger, J., Tehoungue, K., & Omidian, P. A. (2017). "The Opposite of Denial: Social Learning at the Outset of the Ebola Emergency in Liberia." *Journal of Health Communication* 22: 59–65.

Abramowitz, S. A., McLean, K. E., McKune, S. L., Bardosh, K. L., Fallah, M., Monger, J., Tehoungue, K., & Omidian, P. A. (2015). "Community-Centered Responses to Ebola in Urban Liberia: The View from Below." *PLoS Neglected Tropical Diseases* 9: e0003706.

Abrams, L., & Moio, J. (2009). "Critical Race Theory and the Cultural Competence Dilemma in Social Work Education." *Journal of Social Work Education* 45: 245–261.

Adeyi, O. (2018). "Preface." In *Strengthening Post-Ebola Health Systems: From Response to Resilience in Guinea, Liberia, and Sierra Leone*, edited by R. Govindaraj & C. H. Herbst, xi–xii. Washington: World Bank.

Africa Center for Strategic Studies. (2020, April 15). "African Adaptations to the COVID-19 Response." https://africacenter.org/spotlight/african-adaptations-to-the-covide-19-response.

African American Registry (AAREG). "People, Locations, Episode, Krio People of Sierra Leone. A Brief Article." aaregistry.org/story/krio-people-of-sierra-leone-a-brief-article/.

African Spotlight. "The Temne People of Sierra Leone." *Duchess International Magazine*. https://www.duchessinternationalmagazine.com/african-spotlight-the-temne-people-of-sierra-leone/#:-text=Temne,%20are%.

Africana Sankofo. "Kissi People of Sierra Leone, Guinea and Liberia."wordpress.com.

Airhihenbuwa, C. (1995). *Health and Culture: Beyond the Western Paradigm*. Thousand Oaks: Sage Publishers.

Airhihenbuwa, C., Iwelunmor, J., Munodawfa, D., Ford, C., Oni, T., & Agyemang, C. (2020). "Culture Matters in Communicating the Global Response to COVID-19." *PCD Staff* 17: E60.

Alexander, K. A., Sanderson, C. E., Marathe, M., Lewis, B. L., Rivers, C. M., Shaman, J. M., & Eubank, S. (2014). "What Factors Might Have Led to the Emergence of Ebola in West Africa." *PLoS Neglected Tropical Diseases*. http://blogs.plos.org/speakingofmedicine/2014/11/11.

Alie, Joe A. D. (2016). *A New History of Sierra Leone*. Freetown: Blessed Farouk.

Alldridge, T. J. (1901). *The Sherbro and Its Hinterland*. New York: Macmillan and Company, Limited.

Ansumana, R., Bonwitt, J., Stenger, D., & Jacobsen, K. (2014). "Ebola in Sierra Leone: A Call for Action." *The Lancet*. https://doi.org/10.1016/s0140-6736(14)61119-3.

Anya, Oji. (1973). "The Sherbro in the Nineteenth Century – A Coastal People in Transition." MA Thesis, University of Sierra Leone (University of Sierra Leone).

Appiah, K., & Gates, H. (2010). *Africana: The Encyclopedia of the African and African Experience*. Longman, London.

Azevedo, M. (2020). "Ebola Virus Disease Outbreaks and Sustainable Health Security and Economic Development in West and Central Africa." In G*ender and Sustainable Development in Africa*, edited by Maurice N. Amutabi & Elinami V. Sway, 115–134. Nairobi, Kenya: Center for Democracy, Research and Development (CEDRED).

Baize, S., Pannetier, D., Oestereich, L., Rieger, T., Koivogui, L., Magassouba, N., & Günther, S. (2014). «Emergence of Zaire Ebola Virus Disease in Guinea." *New England Journal of Medicine* 371(15): 1418–1425. https://doi.org/10.1056/NEJMoa1404505.

Bangura, Sheka. (2021). *Compelling Lessons from Mano River Union Disasters: A Reflection on Deadly Ebola, Landslides and Floods in Guinea, Liberia and Sierra Leone 2013–17*. Freetown: Sierra Leone Writers Series.

Beah, Ishmael. (2007). *A Long Way Gone: Memoirs of a Boy Soldier*. New York: Sarah Crichton Books.

Bedson, J., Jalloh, M. F., Pedi, D., Bah, S., Owen, K., Oniba, A., Sangarie, M., Fofanah, J. S., Jalloh, M. B., Sengeh, P., & Skrip, L. (2020). "Community Engagement in Outbreak Response; Lessons Learned from the 2014–2016 Ebola Outbreak in Sierra Leone." *BMJ Global Health* 5: e002145.

Bernard, R. (2011a). "Chapter 8: Interviewing I: Unstructured and Semistructured." In *Research Methods in Anthropology*, edited by R. Bernard, 5th ed., 156–186. Lanham: AltaMira Press.

Bernard, R. (2011b). "Chapter 12: Participant Observation." In *Research Methods in Anthropology*, edited by R. Bernard, 5th ed., 256–290. Lanham: AltaMira Press.

Betancourt, J., Green, A., Carrillo, J. E., & Ananeh-Firemponh, O. (2003). "Defining Cultural Competence: A Practical Framework for Addressing Racial/Ethnic Disparities in Health and Health Care." *Public Health Reports* 293–302.

Brach, C., & Frazier, I. (2000). "Can Cultural Competency Reduce Racial Disparities? A Review and Conceptual Model." *Medical Care Research and Review* 57: 181–217.

Branswell, H. (2021). "Bombshell Analysis Traces New Ebola Outbreak to Survivor of West Africa Crisis." Accessed March 2021.

Britannica Online Encyclopedia. *Temne*. https://www.britannica.com/print/article/586495.

Brittian, A. (2015, February 28). "The Fear of Ebola Led to Slayings – And a Whole Village Was Punished." *The Washington Post*. https://www.washingtonpost.com/world/africa/the-fear-of-ebola-led-to-murder-and-a-whole-villiage-was-punished/2015/02/28/a2509b88-a80f-11e4-a162-121d06ca77f1_story.html.

Brown, I., & Daniel, S. (1996). "Disease, Ecology, and Human Behavior." In *Medical Anthropology: Contemporary Theory and Method*, edited by Carolyn Sargent & Thomas Johnson, 183–218. United States of America: Praeger.

Campinha-Bacote, J. (1998). *The Process of Cultural Competenc in the Delivery of Healthcare Services: A Culturally Competent Model of Care*, 3rd ed. Cincinnati: Transcultural C.A.R.E. Associates.

Campinha-Bacote, J. (1999). "A Model and Instrument for Addressing Cultural Competence in Health Care." *Journal of Nursing Education* 8–12.

Campinha-Bacote, J. (2007). *The Process of Cultural Competence in the Delivery of Healthcare Services: A Culturally Competent Model of Care*, 5th ed. Transcultural Care. https://www.transculturalcare.net/Cultural_Competence_Modelhtm.

Campinha-Bacote, J. (2009). "A Culturally Competent Model of Care for African Amricans." *Urologic Nursing* 29: 49–54.

Centers for Disease Control and Prevention: 2014–2016 Ebola Outbreak in West Africa. Accessed October 28, 2020.

Countries and Their Cultures, Germany to Jamaica, Fulani. https://everyculture.com/wc/Germany-toJamaica/Fulani.html.

Cross, T., Bazron, B., Dennis, K., & Issacs, M. (1989). *Towards an Culturally Competent System of Care: A Monograph on Effective Services for Minority Children Who Are Severely Emotionally Disturbed*. Washington: CASSP Technical Assistance Center, Georgetown University Child Development Center.

Diallo, B., Sissoko, D., Loman, N., Bah, H. A., Bah, H., Worrell, M., Conde, I., Sacko, R., et al. (2016). "Resurgence of Ebola Virus Disease in Guinea Linked to a Survivor With Virus Persistence in Seminal Fluid for More Than 500 Days." *Clinical Infectious Diseases. Brief Report. Infectious Disease Society of America.*

Diaz-Cuellar, A., & Evans, S. (2014a). "Diversity and Health Education." In *Cultural Competence in Health Education and Health Promotion*, edited by M. Perez & R. Luquis, 23–58. San Francisco: John Wiley & Sons, Inc.

Diaz-Cuellar, A., & Evans, S. (2014b). "Diversity and Health Education." In *Cultural Competence in Health Education and Health Promotion*, edited by M. Perez & R. Luquis, 2nd ed., 23–58. San Francisco: Jossey-Bass.

Dubois, M., Wake, C., & Sturridge, S. (2020, November 2). "The Ebola Response in West Africa: Explosing the Politics and Culture of International Aid, 2015." https://www.odi.org/publications/9956-ebola-response-west-africa-exposing-politics-culture-international-aid.

Ebola Response Anthropology Platform. (2020, November 30). "Ebola Response Anthropology Platform." http://www.ebola-anthropolgy.net.

Edberg, M. (2013). *Essentials of Health, Culture and Diversity: Understanding People, Reducting Disparities*. Burlington: Jones & Bartlett Publishing.

Encyclopedia Britannica. "Kisi." www.britannica.com/topic/Kisi.

Encyclopedia Britannica. https://www.britannica.com/topic/Vai.

Encyclopedia Britannica. (2017, December 21). https://www.everyculture.com/Ge-It/Guinea.html#ixzz6iN09eZeM.

Fairhead, J. (2014). *The Significance of Death, Funerals, and the After-Life in Ebola-Hit Sierra Leone, Guinea and Liberia: Anthropological Insights into Infection and Resistance*.

Fairhead, J. (2015, April). "Understanding Social Resistance to Ebola Response in Guinea." *Ebola Response Anthropology Platform*. http://www.ebola-anthropology-net/evidence/1269.

Foster, George M. (1998). "Disease Etiologies in Non-Western Medical Systems." In *Understanding and Applying Medical Anthropology*, edited by Peter Brown, 110–117. California: Mayfield Publishing Company.

Fyfe, C. (1964). *Sierra Leone Inheritance*. Oxford: Oxford University Press.

Fyfe, C. (1979). *A Short History of Sierra Leone*, 2nd ed. Addison-Wesley Longman: Longman. Harlow, Ltd.

Fyle, C. M. (1982). *The History of Sierra Leone*. London: Evans Brothers.

Gassel, M. (2014). "How Cultural Norms and Practices Affect Ebola Outbreak." Accessed December 8, 2020. http://publichealth.tufts.edu/About-Us/Public-Health-Rounds-Newsletter/How-Cultural-Norms-and-Practices-Impact-Ebola-Outbreak Page.

Glanz, K., Lewis, F. M., & Rimer, B. K. (1997). "Linking Theory, Research, and Practice." In *Health Behavior and Health Education: Theory, Research, and Practice*, edited by K. Glanz, F. M. Lewis, & B. Rimer, 2nd ed., 19–53. SanFrancisco, CA: Jossey-Vass, Inc.

Goode, T., & Dunne, C. (2003). *Policy Brief 1: Rationale for Cultural Competence in Primary Care*. Washington: National Center for Cultural Competence, Georgetown University Center for Child and Human Development.

Goode, T., & Jones, W. (2004). "Increasing Awareness and Implementation of Cultural Competence Principles in Health Professions Education." *Journal of Allied Health* 29: 241–245.

Gordon, Andrew J. "Cultural Identity and Illness: Fulani Views." researchgate.net.

Greene-Morton, G., & Minkler, M. (2020). "Cultural Competence or Cultural Humility? Moving Beyond the Debate." *Health Promotion Practice* 21: 142–145.

Haken, N., & Fiertz, C. (2020, May 13). "What West Africa's Resilience Can Teach the World About COVID-19: Different Types of Shocks Require Different Types of Capital." *The New Humanitarian*. https://www.thenewhumanitarian.org/opinion/2020/05/13/Fragile-States-Index-West-Africa-coronavirus-resilience.

Hayden, J. (2019). *Introduction to Health Behavior Theory*. Burlington: Jones and Bartlett Publishers.

Heaney, C. A., & Israel, B. A. (1997). "Social Network and Social Support." In *Health Behavior and Health Education: Theory, Research, and Practice*, edited by K. Glanz, F. M. Lewis & B. Rimer, 2nd ed., 179–205. SanFrancisco, CA: Jossey-Vass, Inc.

Hewlett, B. S., & Amola, R. P. (2003, October). "Cultural Contexts of Ebola in Norther Uganda." *Emerging Infectious Diseases* 9(10). http://wwwnc.cdc.gov/eid/article/9/10/02-0493.

Hochbaum, G. M. (1958). *Public Participation in Medical Screening Programs: A Sociological Study*. PHS Publication no, 572. Washington, D.C.: U.S. Government Printing Office.

Holshue, M. L., Debolt, C., & Lindquist, S. (2019). "First Case of 2019 Novel Coronavirus in the United States." *New England Journal of Medicine* 382: 929–936.

Hongoltz-Hetling, M. (2015). "When Science, Faith Clash: In Sierra Leone, a Deadly Gap Between Ritual and Medical Practices." *Valley News*, April 26, 2015.

House, J. S., Umberson, D., & Landis, K. R. (1988). "Structures and Processes of Social Support." *Annual Review of Sociology* 14: 293–318.

Huff, R., & Kline, M. (2007). "The Cultural Assessment Framework." In *Health Promotion in Multicultural Populations: A Handbook for Practitioners and Students*, edited by R. Huff & M. Kline, 2nd ed., 125–145. Thousand Oaks: SAGE.

Idriss, A., Diaconun, K., Zou, G., Senesi, R., Wurie, H., & Witter, S. (2020). "Rural-Urban Health Seeking Behaviours for Non-Communicable Diseases in Sierra Leone." *BMJ Global Health* 5: e002024.

Ijagbemi, E. A. (1977). "Oral Tradition and Emergence of Temne Chiefdoms." *Africana Research Bulletin* (ARB) III(2), March.

Institute of Medicine. (1988). *The Future of Public Health*. Washington, D.C.: National Academy Press.

Jackson, P. (2007). "Reshuffling an Old Deck of Cards? The Politics of Local Government Reform in Sierra Leone." *African Affairs* 106: 95–111.

Jalloh, M., Bunnell, R., Robinson, S., Jalloh, M. B., Barry, A. M., Corker, J., Sengeh, P., VanSteelandt, A., Li, W., Dafae, F., & Diallo, A. A. (2017). "Assessments of Ebola Knowledge, Attitudes and Practices in Forecariah, Guinea and Kambia, Sierra Leone, July–August 2015." *Philosophical Transactions of the Royal Society B: Biological Sciences* 372(1721): 20160304.

James, P. B., Wardle, J., Steel, A., & Adams, J. (2018). "Traditional, Complementary and Alternative Medicine Use in Sub-Saharan Africa: A Systematic Review." *BMJ Global Health* 3(5): e000895. https://doi.org/10.1136/bmjgh-2018-000895.

James, P. B., Wardle, J., Steel, A., & Adams, J. (2019). "Pattern of Health Care Utilization and Traditional and Complementary Medicine Use Among Ebola Survivors in Sierra Leone." *PLoS One* 14(9): e0223068. https://doi.org/10.1371/journal. pone.0223068.

Jones, A. (1981). "Who Were the Vai?" *The Journal of African History* 22(2): 159–178. Accessed December 31, 2020. http://www.jstor.org/stable/181580.

Jones, L. (1994). *The Social Context of Health and Health Care*. Basingstoke: Macmillan.

Joshua Project. "People-in-Country Profile, Kissi, Northern in Sierra Leone, Kissi, Northern in Sierra Leone Ethnic People Profile." joshuaproject.net.

Kanu, M. (2014). "The Ebola Tragedy in West Africa: An Examination of the Sierra Leone Experience and Recommendations for the Future." *Research in Sierra Leone Studies (RISLS): Weave* 2(2): 1–14.

Kanu, M., Baker, E., & Brownson, R. (2008). "Exploring Associations Between Church-Based Social Support and Physical Activity." *Journal of Physical Activity and Health* 5: 504–515.

Kassaye, I. (2015, September 28). "Traditional Healers – Friends or Foes in the Fight Against Ebola?" *UNICE Sierra Leone*. Acccssed November 10, 2020.

Kiefer, C. (2006a). "Chapter 1: Why Anthroplogy?" In *Doing Health Anthropology: Research Methods for Community Assessment and Change*, edited by C. Kiefer, 1–20. New York: Springer Publishing Company, LLC.

Kiefer, C. (2006b). "Chapter 6: The Researcher in and Beyond the Community." In *Doing Health Anthropology: Research Methods for Community Assessment and Change*, edited by C. Kiefer, 80–108. New York: Springer Publishing Company, LLC.

Kleinman, A., Eisenberg, L., & Good, B. (1978). "Culture, Illness, and Care: Clinical Lessons from Anthropologic and Cross-Cultural Research." *Annals of Internal Medicine* 88: 251–258.

Kroeber, A. L., & Kluckhohn, C. (1952). *Culture: A Critical Review of Concepts and Definitions*. Cambridge, MA: Peabody Museum.

Kupferschmidt, K. (2021). "New Ebola Outbreak Likely Sparked by a Person Infected 5 Years Ago." Accessed March 2021.

Lavizzo-Mourey, R., & Mackenzie, E. (1996). "Cultural Competence: Essential Measurements of Quality for Manageed Care Organizations." *Annals of Internal Medicine* 124: 919–920.

Levy, B., & Gaufin, J. (2012). "Practicing Cultural Competence." In *Mastering Public Health: Essential Skills in Effective Practice*, edited by B. Levy & J. Gaugin. Oxford: Oxford University Press.

Like, R. (2011). "Educating Clinicians About Cultrural Comepetence and Dispariries in Health and Health Care." *Journal of Continuing Education in the Health Professions* 31: 196–206.

Little, K. (1949). *The Mende of Sierra Leone*. London.

London School of Hygiene & Tropical Medicine. (2020, November 30). "Grassroots Response to the Epidemic." *Future Learn*. https://www.futurelearn.com/Info/courses/ebola-in-context/0/steps/4843.

Long, T. (2012). "Oviewview of Teaching Strategies for Cultural Competence in Nursing Students." *Journal of Cultural Diversity* 19: 102–108.

Luquis, R. (2014). "Health Education Theoretical Models and Multicultural Populations." In *Cultural Competence in Health Edication and Health Promotion*, 2nd ed., 145–170. San Francisco: John Wiley & Sons, Inc.

Luquis, R., & Perez, M. (2003). "Achieving Cultural Competence: The Challenges for Health Educators." *Journal of Health Education* 34: 131–138.

Luquis, R., & Perez, M. (2014). "Cultural Competency and Health Education: A Window of Opportunity." In *Cultural Competence in Health Education and Health*

*Promotions*, edited by M. Perez & R. E. Luquis, 2nd ed., 293–310). San Francisco: Jossey-Bass.

Luquis, R., Perez, M., & Young, K. (2006). "Cultural Competence Development in Health Educational Professional Preparation Programs." *American Journal of Health Educators*, 37(4): 233–241.

Mackinnon, J., & Maclaren, B. (2012). "Human Resources for Health Challenges in Fragile States: Evidence from Sierra Leone, South Sudan and Zimbabwe." *Journal of Health Economics* 1–18.

Magana, G. D., Kapetshi, J., Berthet, N., Ilunga, B. K., Kabange, F. K., Kingebeni, P. M., & Leroy, E. M. (2014). "Ebola Virus Disease in the Democratic Republic of Congo." *New England Journal of Medicine* 371: 2083–2091. https://doi.org/10.1056/NEJMoa1411099.

Manguvo, A., & Mafuvadze, B. (2015). "The Impact of Traditional and Religious Practices on the Spread of Ebola in West Africa: Time for a Strategic Shift." *The Pan African Medical Journal* 22(Suppl 1): 9. https://doi.org/10.11694/pamj.supp.2015.22.1.6190.

McCann, M., Carter-Pokras, O., Braun, B., & Hussein, C. (2013). "Cultural Competency and Health Literacy: A Guide for Teaching Health Professionals and Students." Universty of Maryland College Park School of Public Health Department of Epidemiology and Biostatistics. https://health.maryland.gov/mhhd/CCHLP/Documents/Cover.pdf.

Middleton, J. (1997). *Encyclopedia of Africa South of the Sahara*, Vol. 4. New York: Charles Scribner's Sons.

Miller, B. (2011). *Cultural Anthropology*, 6th ed. Boston: Prentice Hall.

Ministry of Health and Sanitation. (2015). *Health Sector Recovery Plan, 2015–2020*. Freetown: Ministry of Health and Sanitation, Government of Sierra Leone.

Momodu, S. (2016, July 25). "First Liberia Civil War (1989–19196)." https://www.blackpast.org/global-african-history/first-liberian-civil-war-1989-1996/.

Moon, S., Sridhar, D., Pate, M. A., Jha, A. K., Clinton, C., Delaunay, S., Edwin, V., Fallah, M., Fidler, D. P., Garrett, L., & Goosby, E. (2015). "Will Ebola Change the Game? Ten Essential Reforms Before the Next Pandemic. The Report of the Harvard-LSHTM Independent Panel on the Global Response to Ebola." *The Lancet* 386: 2204–2221.

Nyenswah, T., Kateh, F., Bawo, L., Massaquoi, M., Gbanyan, M., Fallah, M., Nagbe, T. K., Karsor, K. K., Wesseh, C. S., Sieh, S., & Gasasira, A. (2016, February). "Ebola and Its Control in Liberia, 2014–2015." *Perspective* 22(2). Accessed December 2, 2020. www.cdc.gov/eid.

Obermueller, N. M. (2012). "Old Sierra Leonean Remedies Find a Place Alongside Modern Medicine." *International Development Journalism Competition, The Guardian News*.

Oldenburg, B., Hardcastle, D. M., & Kok, G. (1997). "Diffusion of Innovations." In *Health Behavior and Health Education: Theory, Research, and Practice*, edited by K. Glanz, F. M. Lewis, & B. Rimer, 2nd ed., 270–286. SanFrancisco, CA: Jossey-Vass, Inc.

Olukoju, Ayodeji. (2006). *Culture and Customs of Liberia*, 24–147. Westport, CT: Greenwood Publishing Group. ISBN 0313332916. Google Books. Accessed July 24, 2017.

Oosterhoff, P., Mokuwa, E., & Wilkinson, A. (2015). "Community-Based Ebola Care Centres: A Formative Evaluation." http://www.ebola-anthropology.net/case_studies/community-based-ebola-care-centres-a-formative-evaluation.

Paige, R., Jacobs-Cassuto, M., Yershova, Y., & DeJaeghere, J. (2003). "Assessing Intercultural Diversity: An Empirical Analysis of the Intercultural Development Inventory." *International Journal of Intercultural Relations* 27: 467–486.

Penney, J., & Farge, E. (2014, November 20). "Guinea Imam's Trip to Mali Exposes Gaps in Ebola Response." *Reuters*. http://www.reuters.com/article/2014/11/20/us-health-ebola-maliidUSKCN0J42N20141120.

Prochaska, J., Redding, C., & Evers, K. (1997). "The Transtheoretical Model and Stages of Change." In *Health Behavior and Health Education: Theory, Research, and Practice*, edited by K. Glanz, F. M. Lewis, & B. Rimer, 2nd ed., 60–84. SanFrancisco, CA: Jossey-Vass, Inc.

Project Implicit. (2020, October 29). "Take a Test." https://implicit.harvard.edu/implict/takeatest.html.

Psychological First Aid for Ebola. "West African Cultural Norms/Traditions That May Impact Ebola Transmission." Accessed October 2020. http://apps.who.int/iris/bitstream/10665/131682/1/9789241548847_eng.pdf?ua=1.

Richards, P., Amara, J., Ferme, M. C., Kamara, P., Mokuwa, E., Sheriff, A. I., Suluku, R., & Voors, M. (2015). "Social Pathways for Ebola Virus Disease in Rural Sierra Leone, and Some Implications for Containment." *PLoS Neglected Tropical Diseases* 9: e0003567.

Roat, C., Gheisar, B., Putsch, R., & SenGupta, I. (1999). *Cross Cultural Health Care: Bridging the Gap: A Basic Training for Medical Interpreters*. San Francisco: SFCC Press.

Ross, J. S. (1991). "National Library of Medicine, Perinatal Care: The Kuranko Context of Choice." https://pubmed.ncbi.nlm.nih.gov/2022534/.

Schneider, S., & Smith, S. (2021). *Introduction to Public Health*. Burlington: Jones & Bartlett Learning.

Selig, S., Tropiano, E., & Greene-Morton, E. (2006). "Treaching Cultural Competence to Reduce Health Disparities." *Health Promotion Practice* 7: 247S–255S.

Shi, L. and Johnson, J. (2021). Novic Morro's *Public Health Administration: Principles for Population-Based Management*. Burlington, MA: Jones and Bartlett Learning.

Sierra Leone. (2015). "Population and Housing Census National Analytical Report."

Skolnik, Richard. (2021). *Global Health 101*. Burlington, MA: Jones and Bartlett Learning.

Smith and Stephine Davis. (2013). *The Psychologist as Detective*: An Intoduction in Conduting Research in Psychology. Pearson Education, Inc. Boston, MA.

Social Mobilisation Action Consortium. (2020, November 2). "Community-Led Ebola Action (CLEA) Field Guide for Community Mobilisers, 2014." http://restlessdevelopment.org/file/smac-clea-field-manual-pdf.

Sorensen, J., Norredam, M., Dogra, N., Essink-Bot, M., Suumond, J., & Krasnik, A. (2017). "Enhancing Cultural Competence in Medical Education." *International Journal of Medical Education* 8: 28–30.

Spector, R. (2004). *Cultural Diversity in Health and Illness*, 6th ed. Saddle River: Pearson Prentice Hall.

Statistics Sierra Leone (SSL). (2017, October). Accessed December 15. https://www.statistics.sl/images/StatisticsSL/Documents/Census/2015/2015_census_national_analytical_report.pdf.

Statistics Sierra Leone (Stats SL) and ICF. (2019). *Sierra Leone Demographic and Health Survey 2019: Key Indicators*. Freetown and Rockville: Stats SL and ICF.

Steady, F. C. (2011). "The Mano River Union (MRU) and Mano River Women's Peace Network (MARWOPNET)." In *Women and Leadership in West Africa*. New York: Palgrave Macmillan. https://doi.org/10.1057/9781137010391_4.

Strecher, V., & Rosenstock, J. (1997). "The Health Belief Model." In *Health Behavior and Health Education: Theory, Research, and Practice*, edited by K. Glanz, F. M. Lewis, & B. Rimer, 2nd ed., 41–59. SanFrancisco, CA: Jossey-Vass, Inc.

Temne, Encyclopedia Britannica, Encyclopedia Britannica, Inc. (2019, September 16). Accessed January 3, 2021. https://www.britannica.com/topic/Temne.

Terminology, J. C. (2012). "Report of the 2011 Joint Committee on Health Education and Promotion Terminology [Special Supplemental Issue]." *American Journal of Health Education* 1–19.

Tervalon, M., & Murray-Garcia, J. (1998). "Cultual Humility Versus Cultural Competence: A Critical Distintion in Defining Physician Training Outcomes in Multicultural Education." *Journal of Health Care for the Poor and Underserved* 117–125.

Troslair, E. (2020, September 24). "Poverty Facts About Sierra Leone." *Borgen Magazine*. https://www.borgenmagazine.com/facts-poverty-in-sierraleone.

Turnock, B. (2009). *Public Health: What It is and How It Works*, 4th ed. Massachusetts: Jones and Bartlett Publishers.

Tylor, E. B. (1871). *Primitive Culture*, Vol. 1. Mineola, NY: Dover Publication.

Walsh & Oliver Johnson. (2018). *Getting to Zero: A Doctor and a Diplomat on the Ebola Frontline*. London: Zed Books Ltd.

WHO. (2014a). "Ebola Response Team. Ebola Virus Disease in West Africa — The First 9 Months of the Epidemic and Forward Projections." *New England Journal of Medicine* 371(16): 1481–1495. https://doi.org/10.1056/NEJMoa1411100.

WHO. (2014b, October 20). "Nigeria is Now Free of Ebola Virus Transmission." Accessed December 28, 2014. http://www.who.int/mediacentre/news/ebola/20-october-2014/en/.

Wilberforce, D., & Mckee, W. (1886). "Sherbro and the Sherbros; or a Native African's Account of His Country and People [With a Memoir of the Author by W. McKee]."

Wilkerson, A., & Fairhead, J. (2017). "Comparison of Social Resistance to Ebola Response in Sierra Leone and Guinea Suggest Explanations Lie in Political Configurations and Not Culture." *Critical Public Health* 27: 14–27.

Williams, E. (2016, February 3). "Is Cultural Competence Enough?" American Evaluation Association 365 A Tip-a-Day for Evaluators. https://aea365.org/blob/msi-fellowship-week-elizabeth-williams-on-is-cultural-competence-enough.

Winkelman, Michael. (2009). *Culture and Health: Applying Medical Anthropology*. San Francisco: John Wiley and Sons.

World Health Organization. (1992). *Analysis of Questionnaire on Traditional Medicine*. Geneva: World Health Organization. Accessed November 18, 2020 (unpublished document WHO DOC. 5183A/REV. DOC. 6136A).

World Health Organization. (2002). *WHO Traditinal Medicine Strategy 2002 – 2005*. Geneva: World Health Organization. Accessed November 18, 2020. WHO_EDM_TRM_2002.1.pdf.

World Health Organization. (2014a, September). "Ebola Fact Sheet." http://www.who.int/mediacentre/factsheets/fs103/en/.

World Health Organization. (2014b, November 7). "New WHO Safe and Dignified Burial Protocol-Key to Reducing Ebola Transmission." http://www.who.int/mediacentre/news/notes/2014/ebola-burial-protocol/en/.

World Health Organization. (2014c, November 7). "New WHO Safe and Dignified Burial Protocol – Key to Reducing Ebola Transmission." http://www.who.int/mediacentre/news/notes/2014/ebola-burial-protocol/en/.

World Health Organization. (2017). *Atlas of the African Health Statistixs*. Geneva: World Health Organization.

World Health Organization. (2020, September 24). "Sierra Leone." http://www/who.int/countries/sle/en.

Worthington, S. A. (2014, September 24). "Ebola – A Fragile Health Care System's Ripple Effects." Accessed November 11, 2020. http://www.huffingtonpost.com/samuel-aworthington/ebola-a-fragile-healthcar_b_5871080.html.

Yach, D., Mensah, G., Hawkes, C., Epping-Jordan, J., & Steyn, K. (2012). "Chronic Diseases and Risks." In *Global Health: Diseases, Programs, Systems, and Policies*, edited by Michael Merson, Black Robert, & Anne Mills, 3rd ed., 345–407. Burlington, MA: Jones and Bartlett Learning.

# Index

Page references for figures are italicized.

# About the Editors and Contributors

## EDITORS

**Mohamed Kanu** is a professor and former director of the Master of Public Health Program in the Department of Public Health, Health Administration and Health Sciences at Tennessee State University. He received his MPH and PhD from Saint Louis University School of Public Health in St. Louis, Missouri. He also holds an MA degree in Anthropology from the University of Memphis in Memphis, Tennessee.

Dr. Kanu has served as an evaluator and public health consultant for many organizations. He has authored several technical/evaluation reports, peer-reviewed publications, and presented research papers at national, state, and local conferences. He reviews for several scientific journals.

**Elizabeth A. Williams** received her Doctor of Philosophy and Master of Arts degrees in Applied Anthropology with an emphasis in Medical Anthropology from the University of Kentucky (UK). She received her Master of Divinity degree with an emphasis in Ministry and Theology from Vanderbilt University, and a Bachelor of Arts degree in Anthropology from the University of Illinois, Urbana-Champaign.

Dr. Williams additionally holds graduate reading certificates in Behavioral Science and Women's Studies from UK. After receiving her doctorate, Dr. Williams served on the faculty in the Department of Anthropology and Geography at Georgia State University (GSU), as the inaugural Director of Disparity Elimination for the Tennessee Department of Health, and as a senior-level healthcare administrator with the Vanderbilt-Ingram Cancer Center.

Dr. Williams is presently Interim Dean of the College of Public Service and Professor of Public Health in the Department of Public Health, Health Administration and Health Sciences at Tennessee State University in Nashville, TN. She has completed fellowships with the American Evaluation Association, Kellogg Foundation, and Vanderbilt University. In 2010, she was recognized in by Nashville Healthcare Magazine as one of "10 Women to Watch in Healthcare" for her work in health equity, community engagement, and cultural competence.

Dr. Williams is a content contributor to MusiCity Kids, an interactive, social-emotional learning web show for middle school students, and a Provisional Elder in the United Methodist Church.

Noted for her work in eliminating cancer health disparities, cultural competence, community-engaged research, and spirituality/faith and health, Dr. Williams recently authored the book, "Black Women and Breast Cancer: A Cultural Theology," and has published more than a dozen scholarly papers and presented her work to national and international audiences.

**Charles Williams** is Professor Emeritus at the University of Memphis (U of M) in the Department of Anthropology. He received his BA in Social Science from Rust College, and PhD in Anthropology from the University of Illinois. Dr. Williams served as founder and director of the African and African American Studies Program, and the Alcohol and Drug Prevention Research Center (ADPRC) at the University of Memphis. During his career, he has directed research projects dealing with community health, mental health, homelessness, religion, alcohol and drug abuse, HIV/AIDS, and economic development.

Dr. Williams founded the Tennessee Outcomes for Alcohol and Drug Services (TOADS) and was its director until 2000. He also founded and directed the Tennessee Alcohol and Drug Prevention Outcomes Longitudinal Evaluation (TADPOLE), funded by the U.S. Department of Mental Health and Substance Abuse Services, Minority Health TADPOLE, Community-Based TADPOLE, and Tennessee HIV/STD Prevention Evaluation, funded by the Tennessee Department of Health.

Currently, Dr. Williams is a professor and director of the Office of Research and Special Projects and Director of the Roy Wilkins and Earnest A. Smith Institute for Health Equity and Social Justice at Rust College. A community-engaged scholar, Dr. Williams has directed and evaluated youth-focused prevention and leadership programs. He is the author of *African American Life and Culture in Orange Mound: A Case Study of a Black Community in Memphis, Tennessee, 1890-1980*, and has authored several technical/evaluation reports, presented at national, state and local conferences, published in refereed journals and is currently a reviewer for several scientific journals.

## CONTRIBUTORS

**Regina Bash-Taqi** is a public health and education consultant with significant expertise in adolescent health and well-being. She led the development of Sierra Leone's National Strategy for the Reduction of Adolescent Pregnancy and Child Marriage (2018–2022), and the Costed Implementation Plan for Family Planning (2018–2022) with Palladium. She has in-depth knowledge of the Sierra Leone context and is the author of a short guide titled "Policy-Making in Sierra Leone." She has worked as the lead consultant for several studies with organizations, such as ITAD, UNICEF, Christian Aid, Save the Children, and IRC using OECD-DAC evaluation criteria. She is highly skilled in the use of qualitative methods.

**Gloria J. Crawford** has over 25 years experience in ATOD (alcohol, tobacco, and other drugs) in the areas of prevention, data collection, program evaluations, analysis, and management. She has served in the capacities of associate director, research development, evaluator, data manager/administrator, statistician, recorder/transcriber, among other positions, including statistical report writer and editor. As an associate director and liaison to the principal investigator/project director, Alcohol and Drug Prevention Research Center, Department of Anthropology at the University of Memphis, Ms. Crawford's responsibilities included applied and evaluation research related to community health issues, alcoholism, drug prevention and/or abuse, HIV/AIDS, mental health, stroke, hypertension, diabetes, homelessness, religion, mutual aid societies, faith-based organizations, and community development, including providing conferences, workshops, staff/agency trainings and education. Ms. Crawford is a State of Tennessee retiree, and former employee of Rust College, Office of Institutional Research and Assessments, and the Roy Wilkins and Earnest A. Smith Institute, Holly Springs, Mississippi.

www.ingramcontent.com/pod-product-compliance
Ingram Content Group UK Ltd.
Pitfield, Milton Keynes, MK11 3LW, UK
UKHW041843031026
15587UKWH00003B/988

9 781793 645760